Lost and Misunderstood in Psychiatry, but Offering Solutions and Making Resolve

John Peter Veremis

Published by John Peter Veremis, 2020.

Lost and Misunderstood in psychiatry, but Offering Solutions and Making Resolve

By

John Peter Veremis

Original Book printed 2018

John Peter Veremis
Registered Nurse (BSN), Biologist (BSc)
Psychiatric Survivor

LOST AND MISUNDERSTOOD IN PSYCHIATRY, BUT OFFERING SOLUTIONS AND MAKING RESOLVE

First edition. September 11, 2020.

ISBN: 979-8230877288

Written by John Peter Veremis.

Table of Contents

Dedication

I'd like to thank my Psychologist whom I'll call Dr. B for his support in probate court granting me clear victory over oppressive and harmful psychiatry. My battle against psychiatry spanned, (however still fighting its coercion and oppression) over a period of nearly 35 years. I know beyond a shadow of a doubt that eventually I'll win because I'm perfectly healthy mentally and physically always was except for when having side-effects to psychotropic medications (forced onto me, never truly voluntarily), outside influences, and having a "history of mental illness" – placed onto me by gaslighting, incompetent psychiatrists and gaslighting petitioners that wrote false petitions or were written out of malice. I never was given an opportunity to express "my side of the story," due to apathetic, non-empathetic, careless psychiatrists that performed little or no assessment of me as a person or of my "mental health condition." I'd also like to thank my attorney that represented me in probate court making a "formal appearance." My faith in God carried me through the trialing period of psychiatric oppression and harm. I'd also like to thank the priest of my Greek church Fr. Timothy for his prayers.

Preface

I am a family man, enjoy being with my children, significant other, and have many hobbies including: drawing, gardening, riding my bike, and candle making in addition to other mostly arts - crafts and healthy living. I've been a medical professional for nearly 20 years – and still am a Registered Nurse (RN) of nearly 14 years after being a Licensed Practical Nurse (LPN) for 2 years, Mental Health and Direct Care workers for 4 years. I also, take pride in caring for my parents, however my father passed away with hospice from kidney failure three years ago at the age of 86 years. I enjoy reading medical information and am health conscious. I keep mentally, spiritually, and physically healthy by using what I've learned in life's experiences and what makes sense in my learning while reading and studying medical research, social, and religious affairs. I've been involved with the Greek Orthodox Church even as a young boy being in the altar and traveling to nearby cities to help the priest. I was also involved in the Greek dance group, and played Little League baseball for 10 years with 2 of those years being on All-Star teams and most valuable player.

I wrote this book for several reasons and hope the reader becomes inspired in being the best you can be and don't let other people make you think that you're anything less than what you truly believe yourself to be. After all, you're the "captain of your own ship" and know all of your turmoils and triumphs!

This book described personal experiences in mental health over the last 30 years both as a patient and professional offering suggestions to improving the process from family/friendship socializations, petitions to involuntary psychiatric hospitalization in efforts of being better understood and in changing mental health services. I hope this book will inspire you to attain personal growth and help make amends with the mental health system in changing its current practice and viewing the patient as understood and not misunderstood by friends, family, or even psychiatry.

I wrote this book to describe my personal "difficulties" with the field of Psychiatry, but with resolutions which I think will help alleviate unnecessary psychiatric hospitalizations and stressors encountered by mental health patients and staff. It is further hoped that psychiatry no longer will be a "quick fix" for society in treating patients as psychiatrists today carelessly mostly only prescribe medications instead of listening to their patients as was evident in my psychiatric experiences as a patient for nearly 32 years! Patients have reasons for behaving and thinking like they do due to common human needs not being met like personal socialization, food allergies, being listened to and understood, other factors will later be explored during the reading of this book. Psychiatrists today base their "therapy" on medicine without trying to understand the patient. Psychotropic medicine is considered a "quick fix" or band aid covering a sore that doesn't get to the core of the psychiatric issue and each and every time was met with personal opposition. In addition, it saddens me to think that certain family members would rather I be taken away and locked up in a psychiatric hospital then forced to take medicine as opposed to taking the time to listen to what I had to say and trying to understand what I've been trying to convey in resolution of a distraught past. A distraught past with no resolution has caused me to be misunderstood which further caused wrongful psychiatric admissions as felt from personal anguish, stress, and distress.

Chapter One

Inspiration

Writing this book has become truly therapeutic, and hopefully will inspire you to reach your goals, never lose sight of who you really are, and can be. I have been in the psychiatric "arena" for nearly 32 years as a patient, advocate for Human Rights, and as a professional. I carried with me a secret for nearly 32 years that threw me into the realm of psychiatry since my first involuntary psychiatric admission. My secret involved an authoritative figure which influenced future psychiatric "endeavors." Who is this authoritative figure? - The first psychiatrist I ever had. My first psychiatrist stated unprofessional remarks which perpetuated the cycle of me being committed involuntarily time and time again in seeking justice due to his unprofessional remarks. Each involuntary psychiatric admission after the first, revolved around me trying to be heard by someone in the mental health system, community or side-effect to psychotropic medications. I tried telling my story to people within mental health and family, but was left with nothing except mental health professionals and even family thinking that I was delusional, having a psychosis or being hallucinatory. I was involuntarily taken away against my will and placed into a locked in psychiatric unit without my thoughts being explored of as to why I thought what I did each and every time. It seemed as though my concerns also were not taken seriously in the community or even by some of my family as nothing was done regarding my stories of abuse by psychiatry and careless communication in trying to socialize with family and friends until now as in writing this book.

I was a young man and too young to have the last nearly 32 years fought for resolve while trying to forgive and forget the remarks made by an unprofessional authoritative figure – my first psychiatrist. It is difficult to relive the memories of when I tried to break the window in a psychiatric unit in an effort to make the point of how unprofessional the psychiatrist's remarks were and I wasn't sure if the "unsettling" happenings in Detroit were related to the psychiatrist's threatening comment. His unprofessional comment scarred me from early to mid-adulthood which lasted up until I finally found resolve through expressing my thoughts in writing this book, trying to be understood by friends, family, and sessions with my Psychologist. The chair I threw at the window was done in an effort to start a commotion/investigation to make people aware of the psychiatrists' threatening remark, and because of the "unsettling" experiences I had while in Detroit, however I never felt "paranoid." A side-effect that I had on a forced psychotropic medication – Haldol (25 years ago) was me "hearing a voice" telling me "I'm the head of the FBI." I entered the Saginaw Township Police Department after hearing the hallucination and asked to speak with someone. I then again said "I'm the head of the FBI." The office attendant then said "I believe you." This real-life story is significant, because as discovered through therapy with my Psychologist, it was determined that the "FBI story" was just a story, because I wanted the psychiatrists that never took the time to know me as a person and misdiagnosed me to be arrested.

Picture if you will, a young man in his early 20s living in Detroit 1990 away from friends and family and in a big city overnight for the first time. I remember a housemate telling me how he dodged bullets trying to pick up patients as an emergency medical technician. Detroit has changed for the better since 1991 with new condominiums and flower beds along main downtown streets. I believe the stigma and reputation of the part of Detroit I lived in nearly 32 years ago unfortunately, casted negative thoughts in my mind while I was living there. I recently visited Detroit and was impressed with the new downtown architecture and social gatherings surrounding the center of the city.

The big city culture was too impersonal for me for the first few weeks while living in Detroit nearly 32 years ago when I was 20 years old. Although I enjoyed the busy cars and crowds at Hart's Plaza – downtown, I also missed the quiet smaller city life I experienced in my hometown. I needed a break from the new city I had been a recent inhabitant of, felt as though there was a kind of harassment in the locker room of a gym at Wayne State University (WSU) and called my parents for a ride back to my home town for a brief visit back home.

I arrived back to my home town in Saginaw, MI after calling my parents to take me back to a familiar environment so that I could rest. I needed somewhere familiar, because I felt consumed by the big city life and its culture. My dad and uncle requested to me that I see a therapist, but none were available at that time at night – later in the evening. Instead, we visited the psychiatric unit at a local hospital and met a doctor whom I will call Dr. "X" for the sake of legal and ethical considerations. I was tired and asked the psychiatrist "so what kind of treatment, how are you going to treat me?" He responded by directly and wholeheartedly telling me "I'm going to shoot you in the head." I calmly went back to my room, picked up a chair and attempted to throw it through the window – I wanted to make the point that the psychiatrist was unprofessional in saying what he did and most importantly to start a commotion hoping it would lead to an investigation to what the psychiatrist said. In addition, I felt uneasy with the "harassment I felt while in the locker room at WSU and asked myself was the threatening comment I experienced by the psychiatrist related to the harassment I felt in the locker room? I never really believed he would "shoot" me, but thought to myself how wrong and unprofessional for him to say. No, I didn't hallucinate what the psychiatrist had said – I know what that's like. I hallucinated only while taking certain psychotropic medications after starting my psychiatric mental health experiences. Other times hallucinations occurred while tapering off certain psychotropic medications too quickly as the mind needs time to overcome the effects of the medication. I remember the first medicines Dr. "X" put me on nearly 33 years ago – Stelazine and Loxitane which made my shoulders cramp and Haldol which made me feel like a robot zombie while hallucinating as side-effects. Why would Dr."X" mention what he did – the unprofessional remarks? I'm not sure, but I carried his unprofessional remarks a secret until now.

I enjoyed being a student at Wayne State University in Detroit. The university had so much to offer including many fields of interest. I ultimately graduated with a Bachelor's of Science degree in Biology and a member of the Golden Key National Honor Society from Wayne State University. It wasn't until nearly fifteen years later when I received my second and third degrees of associate's then Bachelor's degrees in Nursing as a Licensed Practical and Registered Nurse at other colleges and universities.

I explored the city life while living in Detroit. Student housing near campus was nearly non-existent at the time when I was living there. Most of the students commuted to classes. There was much to do including visiting the ball park and coffee houses. I particularly enjoyed taking the transit bus to downtown Detroit. I visited restaurants, stores, and parks while exploring downtown. Most of all, I visited the university's library and was often the first one there and the last to leave. I remember studying many hours a day when I wasn't in class. Even though I was busy with school, I still found time to work-out for exercise. I learned how to cook basic meals, but mostly ate at local restaurants. I enjoyed the ethnic backgrounds of the city and tried many different foods. The University Center had restaurants and resources available for students. I was a part of the student life by tutoring various subjects such as Biology, Chemistry, and Physics. I also participated in other work-study programs for an additional extra income. The extracurricular work-study experiences I had included were working at football games where I helped sell tickets and seat the crowd. I eventually enjoyed the big city life and made some friends, but devoted my life to mostly studying and getting good grades while at Wayne State University after my return from home.

I pursued graduate school after my undergraduate study at Wayne State University in 1995 for a year then returned back to my home town after once again having an "unsettling" experience with my roommate and graduate studies. I was in search of employment and decided to apply to a company I'll call "Y," (due to legal issues) as a laboratory technician. I also applied to the Michigan Department of Civil Services, Laboratory Assistant position where I received Band 01. I called the Dep't of Civil Service to find out what Band 01 meant as

I spoke to a lady I'll name as Mrs. G due to confidentiality. I asked Mrs. G "What does band 01 mean" and she said "You're first in line for an interview" I then asked her "Where do I go for an interview?" she said "You got the highest score." – an informal interview . I applied to company "Y" through a contracting company – the same company I worked before. The contracting company found another job for me at company "Y" in the same department but in a different building. I unfortunately was "let go" by company "Y" without explanation and was even threatened by whom appeared to be my supervisor.

I began picketing company "Y," sending flyers, and placing them under windshield wipers, because I wanted the public to be aware that I was threatened, wrongfully discharged and sought for resolve. I made several attempts to seek justice of the threats made against me while working at company "Y" by going to the city police department and company offices. As I mentioned before, I can compare a hallucination to real living because I hallucinated while taking Haldol – and I knew I did. In addition, I was not paranoid in the threat but wanted resolve to what occurred and wrongful discharge.

I found hallucinations very different. I never hallucinated or was delusional before taking first generation psychotropic medications. The psychotropic first generation medications caused additional side-effects of making me lethargic and catatonic at times. I often described my experiences while on first generation psychotropic medications as having "difficult dreams" in the daytime. It wasn't until several different attempts at trying new medications as I was forced through a court order to take - that I found medications that didn't cause me to hallucinate, be delusional, or have abnormal involuntary muscle movements except when coming off of them too quickly without tapering. I adamantly denied psychotropic medications because I believe in the power of talk therapy either with a therapist or socializing and finding the root cause of psychosis, delusions, and hallucinations which may be due to allergies to foods, inadequate sleep, unresolved situations from the past, and even psychotropic medication side effects! It was apparent that psychiatrists labeled me as being a paranoid schizophrenic to bill insurance companies which later led to court orders keeping me on the medications and forced treatment.

I tried explaining my story to mental health professionals, and psychiatrists after pick-up orders, unfortunately wasn't resonantly heard and was once again committed into psychiatric hospitals all stemming from two family members which hardly ever communicated with me and even lived an hour and a half away! Each time I began my picketing or flyer protests, I was met with police officers, and petitions to take me for psychiatric evaluation. Here I am 33 years later still protesting, but have learned to make a more civil appearance, write a book rather than flyers or picket signs. I've tried to break from the psychiatric system, but seemed as though each time I tried I was met with more resistance until now as in expressing myself in writing this book and meeting people on social media with experiences similar to mine. I'm once again on a treatment order where I'm forced to take psychotropic medications or be taken back to an inpatient psychiatric hospital for injections.

Thirty three years later, and I have not made much progress in overcoming the feelings I have for psychiatrist Dr. "X" or the incident that happened at company "Y". It makes me sad and even frustrated knowing that a field of medicine –psychiatry supposedly devoted to helping the mind and spirit has caused so much misunderstanding, anguish, stress, duress in my life and caused our family to split. Where was the talk therapy that I requested? Unfortunately, even members of my family lacked adequate talk and socialization with me which further made for creeping petitions for a "psychiatric evaluation" which inevitably ended up with me being an inpatient in a psychiatric hospital on and off for nearly 32 years. Instead, I was forced to take medications which I vehemently protested in taking and which produced detrimental side-effects.

The incidences with my psychiatrist doctor "X" and company "Y" are being resolved. I'm now writing a book to help vent my frustrations and find closure to a time in my life which was unjust and consumed most of my adult life to this point. A mind with no resolve tries to find closure in ways that don't necessarily harm it or is even ill. The mind responds to stressors in many ways and if there's no resolve it actually may become delusional, have a psychosis or experience hallucinations – a normal response to years of abuse.

I suffered mental anguish and duress for years and for years my mind wanted to believe I was involved in an out of court case settlement. It was my only hope and sanctity at the time to believe I was being heard. Would anyone listen?

There was once an incident which happened and could prove to my psychiatrists, that I'm far from being paranoid and the only times I hallucinated were on psychotropic medications. I remember back in 2005 I was sitting in the garden where I worked as a mental health worker and noticed a man lying on the ground near a window in the psychiatric unit of which I found out he tried to escape. I was on break, but followed the man whom turned out was an ex-customs officer at six foot four and 250 pounds. He began running through a ditch then fields of tall grass. I followed him while dialing 911 emergency on my phone. A helicopter was sent to the fields where I chased the patient.

The ex-customs agent told me "Don't come near me, stay away." I did just that, but chased him with my phone and gave directions to the helicopter which was now headed our direction. The police officers captured the ex-customs agent and brought him back to the mental health unit without any harm to the patient or officers. That was a true occasion - I reacted to an emerging situation by going after the ex-customs agent patient. That incident proved to myself and other people that cared to listen, that I'm not paranoid by any means, but ethical and moral in doing the right thing. The patient was brought back to the mental health unit safely.

The incident of chasing the patient occurred while I worked as a mental health worker at a local area's hospital behavioral/psychiatric unit. I chose to work as a mental health worker because sociology and mental health were interests of mine since the first day I stepped foot into a psychiatric hospital – even as a patient. I further enjoyed being a mental health worker to positively change mental health after being personally negatively involved in mental health as a patient. While a patient back in 1991 there was a young African American man that influenced me to attend groups and seek spiritual guidance which was a positive experience among the mostly all negative I personally experienced while an inpatient in psychiatric units.

There was an additional time which allowed me to gain confidence in mending my situation as when I applied to the Civil Service Department as a Laboratory Scientist Assistant, after I completed my Bachelor's of Science degree in Biology from Wayne State University in 1995. I remember sending my application to the State Department then receiving a letter back stating Band 01. I called the State Department to inquire what "Band 01" meant and spoke to a lady whom I'll remain confidential and she said that Band 01 meant I was "first in line for an interview." I, then asked her "Where do I go for an interview?" and she said "You got the highest score." Interesting that I had no formal interview, yet received the highest score. This conversation occurred near the time that I applied to company "Y" – before being harassed, threatened and wrongfully discharged. I was confident of my abilities.

I've noticed the good and bad in all of my experiences being a psychiatric patient. I often said to myself if ever there was a reason for me to be involuntarily committed so many different times in a psychiatric unit was to arrest psychiatrists and change psychiatry forever! I truly enjoyed working in the mental health profession. In fact, I had a job waiting for me as a nurse practitioner in mental health, but was withdrawn from the graduate program only weeks before graduation for dispersing flyers of my protest of company "Y" at my clinical site – again a non justifiable reason for discharge. The flyers focused on trying to find resolve with company "Y" – 18 years later. I realize 18 years past is a long time, but my mind needed resolve before I could move onto the next stage in my life. I have since then developed coping strategies which allowed me to better understand the circumstances of what happened while working in company "Y" and remarks by doctor "X". In addition, I can recognize when having a delusion and hallucination of which both happened while I was taking psychotropic –first generation medications and while being weaned off of them. I no longer take the medications which caused me to have delusions and hallucinations.

Something interesting that I discovered also during the last 20 years was the fact that some flavorings in certain foods were linked to causing hallucinations in people as described by a news show I had seen then. It was interesting to note that I stopped eating the certain potato chips which aired the concern of possible hallucinations caused by their product and felt better physically but never hallucinated while eating the chips. I can't link the chips with certain additives to causing me hallucinations, but it helps to understand that sometimes the foods we eat may trigger an allergic like response which in some people may cause them to hallucinate.

I read material and follow concerns so that I lead a healthy lifestyle. I try to eat foods that won't affect my body in causing heart disease or weight gain. I also, believe in living as natural as can be without medications. That's another reason why I detest being placed on medications – especially involuntarily. I enjoy being a part of the medical profession because I can encourage healthy living and care for people needing assistance to live healthy lives. I also appreciate, and understand certain medications such as for diabetes and hypertension etc. may be required in overcoming various physical diseases.

The mental health profession allowed me to stretch my creativity and work ethics. Although I was a patient in mental health, I've also always enjoyed working as a mental health professional and nurse. I'm an avid worker and enjoy designing and starting new programs. It was rather unique for me to work in a mental health unit being a patient there a few years prior to starting my work. I started many group discussions and created new groups and activities for the patients. I seemed to find the loop holes and improved on the ways groups were presented which involved the patients and staff leading discussions. The management at the hospital's behavioral unit I worked at quickly recognized my good work ethics and placed me in various committees to use me as a reference in problem solving. I remember starting a Wellness group and added to Focus, and Agenda groups. I was even on the psychiatric's new building committee. My group experiences involved both the adult and adolescent side of the behavioral/psychiatric unit. The Wellness group was one of my proudest groups as I originated it at the psychiatric hospital where I worked and was a patient of years prior. I enjoyed encompassing in the Wellness group holistic methods including the major aspects of life such as spirituality, leisure, self, environmental, nutritional, and physical. I was flexible in group discussions teaching new material and trying to include each patient. I also encouraged other workers to lead group discussions on the days I didn't work. I received many company praises and was involved in meetings which easily could have led to advancement in hospital administration.

I knew in my heart that I was much more than any psychiatrist diagnosed me as being or mental health worker wrote hastily conjured on their papers to keep me in the inpatient psychiatric hospital another day. Aside from the wrongful inpatient psychiatric hospitalizations, I had to deal with stigma and stereotyping in the "outside" world of having "mental illness." People that knew I was hospitalized were quick to initially judge my mental health, but soon changed their minds when they started talking to me or heard of all my accomplishments.

Working in the psychiatric unit which I was a patient of, didn't affect me too much, because I knew the circumstances which caused me to be committed involuntarily and knew I was above any diagnosis. In fact, I showed one of the workers the room I stayed in while a patient there nearly 10 years prior to working there. I was comfortable in having people learn I was a patient in the psychiatric unit which later was a place I worked, because I knew I truly never needed to be there - I was never a threat to myself, or anyone else. The "reason" for being admitted at the time I described to the other worker was because I was "catatonic" as described by a family member and needed a medication adjustment which again didn't truly meet criteria and was taking the medicine from a court order for involuntary psychiatric hospitalization, but I knew that everything about me was fine except for side-effects to psychotropic medications and having an unresolved distraught past. I knew the catatonia wasn't normal, but I also knew it was a side-effect from a psychotropic medication I was taking at the time, because I never experienced it before taking the medication. The catatonic state felt as though my brain had frozen. I knew what was happening in my environment while I was catatonic, but had no interests in interacting with anyone. I felt as though I was in a very relaxed mind set, but had no affinity in communicating with anyone.

I know myself as being a very intelligent person with two Bachelor's degrees one in Nursing and the other in Biology. I nearly completed my Family Nurse Practitioner degree. In fact, I walked across the stage during the graduate ceremony and as a member in an International Nurses' Honor Society. I was nearly ready to graduate and carried a 3.9 GPA on a 4.0 scale towards my Family Nurse Practitioner degree in graduate school. In addition to my academic achievements and scholarships, I've also starred as a most valuable player two years in the North Little League. I enjoy sports and am the kind of person that can do well at nearly any kind of sport. I am good with my hands, and enjoy drawing, bowling, playing ping-pong, and gardening. I also learn quickly and help repair appliances and building structures of my parent's five rental houses.

I hope you gain inspiration while reading this book and never let anyone tell you you're something that in your heart you know not to be true. Too many times people have tried to belittle me, were condescending and even tried undermining me but each time, I knew better. The next chapter will focus on the petition which unfortunately, for me was the beginning of many needless inpatient psychiatric hospitalizations which lead to involuntary admissions based on being misunderstood. I chose petition as being an early chapter in my book, because so much of my life revolved around mental health, and a petition was the first step that got me committed involuntarily into a psychiatric unit needlessly each time next to nearly non-existent and even ineffective communication with family and friends. Each time I fought the system and told every listening person that I was healthy but needed for someone to listen to me so that I can express my feelings and thoughts and you know what? I can pick the honest and empathetic workers out from the ones that conjure ideas in making me look like I required psychiatric assistance for billing purposes etc. I learned quickly that inpatient psychiatric hospitals are also like businesses fighting to make evidence for a person to stay another day even if it meant stretching the truth to make the "patient" seem "crazy." I know of some statements that were written down by mental health professionals describing myself were inaccurate but based on my prior "history of being committed." I can honestly say that I feel like a litmus test as I did during my first involuntary psychiatric hospitalization nearly 33 years ago, and can seek an honest mental health worker/ professional including doctors from the ones that try to sabotage my character to make me look like I required "another day" in the psychiatric hospital for billing purposes.

Each of my inpatient psychiatric hospitalizations could have been cared for at home or a Soteria house. I knew the culprits of each "bazaar" behavior such as distributing flyers for resolve everywhere I went for years. My behaviors centered around side-effects from first generation psychotropic medications and unresolved negative situations. Psychotropic medications are mind altering medications. They affect brain chemicals known as neurotransmitters. A medication that produces too much of an affect may actually cause the undesired response. Patients sometimes hallucinate, have psychosis, and are delusional while on psychotropic medications and may be even coming off the medication, if not tapered appropriately. First generation psychotropic medications have more common side-effects than the second generational ones. Sleep is an important aspect of brain health. Inadequate amounts of sleep make the brain dream during the day sometimes in what could be considered a delusion or hallucination. A delusion is a belief by the person which to the ordinary person is determined not to be true. A hallucination can involve visual, olfactory, tactile, or hearing senses. The factor of poor eating may be related to possible food allergies or poor nutrition leading to unhealthy habits which may also inadvertently cause delusions and/or hallucinations. Unresolved negative incidences in people's lives need to be resolved or may come back in different forms as delusions or hallucinations in efforts to resolve them.

Chapter Two

Petition Process

A person being petitioned into a psychiatric hospital must meet the criteria of either being a threat to themselves or someone else. Anyone can petition an individual into a psychiatric hospital, if the above criteria are met or in my case being misunderstood and or influenced by "paranoid" family or medical staff. After a petition is written, it is presented before a judge then to the police department for a pick-up order. The police then pick-up the alleged "mentally ill" individual, and take him or her to the emergency room to be evaluated by a doctor. The doctor then will determine, if the person requires inpatient psychiatric hospitalization and is medically cleared. The nuance, however is that the doctor will in mostly, sign the person into the psychiatric hospital, because the community "fears" having an alleged "mentally ill" person on the streets with a "prior history" as from the stigma of "mental illness." In addition, the emergency room is most always busy thus making for an evaluation by the ER doctor a moot circumstance, because the doctors have no time but send the patient to the psychiatric hospital after medical clearance as to the only reasons I can personally attest.

The petition process makes sense in practicality and in a perfect world may work, however human emotions and the public fear of the unknown in mental health makes the petition process unfavorable for a truly healthy person, but with a "mental health history." The petition process is often times met with hospital staff in a busy ER that don't have time to determine if a person is truly mentally ill and is a threat to himself or herself. The ER doctor often times will base their determination of psychiatric admission on the individual's history or petition as I've personally witnessed many times.

Reality is as found through my personal experiences of being petitioned then involuntarily committed into a psychiatric hospital as being unjust, unfair, and caused me, close family and friends mental anguish, duress, and distress. I have found that psychiatry is mostly based on hearsay and may even involve individuals starting a petition process out of ignorance in truly what I was thinking and/or malice. Isn't psychiatry supposed to help the individual person of being alleged "mentally ill?" What if a person refuses to be admitted into a psychiatric hospital because they "feel fine," but are misunderstood or the victim of "paranoid" individuals not interested in even trying to communicate with the alleged mentally ill individual as was my case? Because, I was never a threat to myself or anyone else, I could have been "treated" in the comfort of my own home or at a therapist's office. In addition, Soteria houses – as used in various parts of the world would have been a benefit (Soteria houses can be used for all mental health condition patients and will be described in greater detail in Chapter Six.) Thirty long days is an average length of stay in a psychiatric hospital, if involuntarily committed as I personally experienced. Any amount of time spent involuntarily in a psychiatric hospital was not welcomed by me and far too long of a period of time away from family, friends, and work.

Each pick up order that had me taken to the ER for evaluation led me to being involuntarily admitted into a psychiatric hospital, but why? I was never a threat to myself, or anyone else. The gray area as with my most recent involuntary hospitalization lies in my behavior of distributing flyers and/or picketing a company to make a point for my Rights of freedom of speech and justice. Again, the ER doctors were faced with either committing me or not into a psychiatric hospital. They generally error on "being safe" and have me committed into the hospital as are their thoughts of being "paranoid." How it affects me is that I once again, fall through the cracks of not meeting criteria to be admitted but am committed based on the ER doctor's thoughts of "being safe" and a petitioner that never took the time to talk to me and find out what I was truly thinking.

The petition process unfortunately, has many loop holes that involve human emotions of professionals making haste decisions which affect the lives of those being petitioned. The petition process must also ask the question of how does the alleged "mentally ill" person feel or thoughts they have? After all, it's how the person understands their own mind and body which should matter the most in caring for an alleged "mentally ill" individual. Should doctors intervene and have the person involuntarily committed into a psychiatric hospital if the individual says they feel fine, and are not a threat to themselves, or someone else? I think not, the doctors may refer that person to a therapist or Psychologist if the person desires, but I know commitment into a psychiatric hospital involuntarily is not the right answer.

The entire process of involuntarily admitting someone into a psychiatric hospital starts with the petition. What of the alleged "mentally ill" individual? I was most recently placing flyers under windshield wipers stating my concerns of what happened to me while working at company "Y" when I was taken into the back seat of a police car then to ER for psychiatric evaluation. I refused medications while at the hospital to make the point that I didn't need to be there, but instead required a good attorney to sue Dr."X" and company "Y." Each involuntary admission resulted in me going in front of a judge explaining why I didn't need to be in the hospital, but each time the judge sided with the doctor which based his or her decision on my "history," petitioner comments, behavior, and the legal and medical profession "playing it safe" for the community. I don't object to being safe, but not in jeopardy of my Rights.

The last visit was worse than the rest. I had to wait for the judge in an actual jail cell! – I committed no crime and they even transported me to and from the hospital in handcuffs with shackles on my feet and in a police car! I lost all my Rights and was actually treated like a criminal! After I arrived back to the psychiatric hospital, staff apologized saying I didn't need to be in a jail cell. Where was my freedom of speech? The stigma of mental health led me to being treated like a criminal. I was soon transported back to the psychiatric hospital with a court order to be treated. I purposely refused to take medications before the hearing to make the point that I felt comfortable with who I was, and was not a threat to myself or anyone else. I felt good in who I was and was functional in carrying out my daily activities and still helped my medically frail parents. I made the decision to not work during the time I distributed flyers, because I wanted some time off for doing what I had wanted to do and complete graduate school before the petitioner stated that because I wasn't working she would have me committed again (wrongfully).

I often woke up at three in the morning to study for my tests and complete class assignments. My studies were early in the morning so that I could spend time with my family and send my son to his school. I enjoyed studying for my graduate Family Nurse Practitioner classes and contributed every day in classroom discussions. My graduate school was put on hold but was withdrawn from the program soon after being hospitalized. I was later court ordered to take medication and was forced once again to take the second generation medication I had been taking just a few years prior to my last hospitalization. I currently have the side-effects of cotton like dry mouth, weight gain, and occasional involuntary eyelid and hand muscle movements.

The petition and hospitalization took my freedom away and caused mental anguish, duress, and stress through being hospitalized involuntarily into a psychiatric hospital for 30 days - again. A person with a previous history of being admitted into a psychiatric hospital of which he/she was admitted involuntarily and even with misunderstood pretenses is vulnerable to being admitted again and again, because of their "history," if there is no resolve of past situations. How do I know? It happened to me, again and again! I felt as though I had to become more vocal in letting the psychiatric community know my discourse in the process from petition to being involuntarily committed into a psychiatric hospital. I've let many people in the mental health profession and public offices know of changes that need to be made in mental health and am still waiting for their reply. I will not end my struggles in mental health until more people are aware of the carelessness of how my Rights were taken away by a system that requires to be more empathetic and basis their "therapy" on the quick fix of psychotropic medications and their own thoughts of "paranoia" wondering If I'm "safe" or not.

It is too easy for the ER doctor to check a box stating the person is "mentally ill," therefore requiring hospitalization in an inpatient psychiatric unit. The "box" the doctor checks basically is related to a paragraph stating that the person is declared "mentally ill" and may cause harm to themselves or someone else. The statement "box" is located as part of the "medical evaluation." I object to the statements in the "box," because I was never a threat to myself or anyone else, but carried the stigma of being declared "mentally ill," which unfortunately stereotyped me as being a threat. The stigma of being "mentally ill" makes me vulnerable to the mental abuse of being thought of as a threat to myself and someone else which would have me committed into a psychiatric hospital again many times. This vicious cycle of being declared "mentally ill" therefore, a threat to myself or someone else has ruined parts of the last 30 years of my life through involuntary commitments into psychiatric hospitals, forced medications, and outpatient therapy sessions.

Let's explore why the ER doctor may be pressured into checking the box which inevitably commits someone into a psychiatric hospital. What if the doctor decided not to commit someone into a psychiatric hospital after a petition and the alleged mentally ill individual committed a crime after released from ER? The doctor may be held accountable for not committing the alleged mentally ill individual into a psychiatric hospital. Therefore, the doctor errors on "being safe" – protecting his/her medical license and commits the person into a psychiatric hospital. The right to sue by the individual falsely committed into a psychiatric hospital is evident, but will "be a waste of time and money" as stated by an attorney of which I sought in retributions for medical malpractice and wrongful placement against my will into many psychiatric hospitals. So you see, doctors believe they must commit someone into a psychiatric hospital and face little consequences for admitting a "heathy" individual, if a petition is put in order. Doctors may ultimately be held accountable, if the alleged mentally ill individual actually hurt themselves or someone else, and were not hospitalized into a psychiatric unit after a psychiatric evaluation.

I personally witnessed these kinds of needless hospitalizations many times, recently related to my ways of practicing freedom of speech leading to decisions by ER doctors that I was not taking psychotropic medications, therefore allegedly not thinking clearly. Even if that were true, these were no reasons to have me committed into a psychiatric hospital. The mental health diagnosis placed on me was in itself also wrong as self-proclaimed which added more reason for me not to take the psychotropic medications. Psychiatry has been difficult for me, because its gone against my own feelings and thoughts of how I wanted to deny ingesting medications which caused side-effects and personal freedom to live how I want to live aside from stigma of being mislabeled "mentally ill."

Psychiatry has left me with few individuals within the system of which I believe to have a truly empathetic ear. My struggle within the mental health system is real because too few mental health professionals are compassionate and empathetic to a maltreated individual by psychiatric professionals. I'm willing to forgive Doctor "X" and company "Y," but psychiatry needs to be changed. Psychiatry needs to focus more on the individual patient and realize talk therapy is important to some people as compared to medication or any other forms of therapy.

The reason for me being readmitted again and again in psychiatric hospitals was my approach for closure by placing flyers under people's windshield wipers describing my concerns with Doctor "X" and company "Y" – not finding resolve, and being misunderstood often times not even tried to be understood by certain family or psychiatry. In addition, the stigma of being considered "mentally ill" sets up the possibility of once again being admitted against my will in a psychiatric hospital. I believe the root cause to my hospitalizations were related to first generation psychotropic medications, being misunderstood and trying to find resolve from heinous past experiences.

The anecdote to the system requires something practical and without making health professionals accountable in a way that jeopardizes the freedom of speech or personal life of an alleged mentally ill person. Being admitted frequently into psychiatric hospitals have caused much stress for the obvious reasons of being taken away against my own will and losing my Rights as a person.

The time away from my family was obviously a concern with each involuntary admission. I missed my children especially, while being admitted into the hospital. I had custody of my son towards his most recent years and he lives with me. He's 21 years old now and we live nearly a mile from my parents whom he could visit for support. My daughter lives with her mother from another marriage.

Each hospitalization started the same with me questioning why I was there. I was mostly to myself for the first few nights while in the hospital as a way to sort of vent my frustrations. I was hardly in the mood to speak with anyone to describe why I may have been there. Eventually I opened up more, and began participating in group discussions. I enjoyed participating in groups, and often had things to say that I felt helped other people which were hospitalized. I learned to be empathetic and had a good listening ear in making people feel better of themselves and in their understanding of certain life's occasions. I often thought to myself "What could I do so that being involuntarily committed into a psychiatric hospital doesn't happen again?" I tried to logically think what I could do to prevent another hospitalization, but I knew deep down inside that I had to make resolve with Dr." X," company "Y," psychiatry, and be better understood by family and friends.

Although the process of being committed into a psychiatric hospital begins with a petition something must be done with how easy it is for someone to write a petition. I was involuntarily committed into a psychiatric hospital many times, and often wondered how the petitioner would act, if they were petitioned into a psychiatric hospital involuntarily. True, I perhaps may have acted eccentrically at times with bazaar ways of expressing my frustrations by using flyers, but knew I never needed to truly be hospitalized.

The petition is the first paper that starts the process of committing someone into a psychiatric hospital. The petition should be presented to the petitioner with a paper stating legal reasons to actually have someone petitioned attached with it. A document describing legal reasons for petitioning should be a part of the petition in clarifying the actual legal role of the petition. In addition, the person being petitioned should have the option of seeking a therapist and or Psychologist, if they desired before the process of "psychiatric evaluation" is carried out. I mention a paper required for actual reasons to petition, because how else and why was I petitioned? Perhaps the petitioner would think twice to justify, if the person actually needed to be petitioned into a psychiatric hospital. A paper that clearly describes legal reasons for petitioning someone will explore other options such as a list of references that could be used in place of a hospitalization. These references may include addresses to Soteria houses, therapist, Psychologist, or drop-in shelter for the mental health condition individual.

The petition is a powerful piece of paper which unfortunately many times starts the lengthy path of hearsay and common fears of the unknown. Medical professionals are nearly forced into complying with a petitioner merely to prevent a backlash of possibly the alleged "mentally ill person going off in society and actually causing harm to themselves or someone else and "being safe."

We must also consider the person that's being petitioned. I'm rather laid back, easy-going and friendly-nice. A person that may be a "higher strung out" individual or not willing to be passive would be less apt to be petitioned, because they may voice their opinion more resonantly except for extremely disgruntled individuals. Therefore, I believe my personality may have set me up to be admitted several times. People know me as being a person to take the punches as they come and have the "patience of a saint" as stated by a fellow nurse.

Writing this book once again may help express my feelings even to the petitioner(s) and eventually cause amends with them. I believe in "forgetting," forgiving, and letting go, but justice in karma – what comes around goes around has been also thought of. I don't hold many grudges. If I do hold a grudge, I usually forgive the person when the time is right. The other aspect of the petition could be that of malice. I believe a petitioner may at times write the petition in a manner in order to inflict grief for the person being petitioned. I mention malice as an intent, because that possibility must also be examined and explored due to a system that already leaves individuals with a mental health history vulnerable to being committed again inappropriately.

My natural tendencies are to amend a situation and that is what I think makes me a good nurse in my professional life. What can we do to help the system so that it actually helps people that need help and is not abusive to people such as myself that would do well with outpatient therapy which never truly required inpatient psychiatric hospitalizations? I believe education is important and should start first with those petitioning. The petitioner should be presented with papers to review as to the actual reasons for petitioning someone into a psychiatric hospital. The petitioner may then determine that the person doesn't qualify to be petitioned, but instead just needs a re-direction. For instance, the petition may be presented with telephone numbers of local 24 hour drop-in shelters for homeless people or maybe even a 24 hour hot-line for suicidal or lonely people. The petitioner could then make the alleged emotionally distraught person aware of the community services. In addition, the petitioner may already be aware of a therapist or Psychologist that is consoling with the alleged emotionally distraught individual and either encourage the person see the therapist/Psychologist or have the therapist/Psychologist see the person that may be petitioned. Communication between the petitioner and the alleged emotionally distraught individual should be apparent, if possible. Community resources with counseling hotlines should be attached to the petition papers. Then as a last resort, the petitioner may consider the final say of actually petitioning someone.

Another force that will bring light to the petition process is greater public awareness that not everyone petitioned is truly emotionally distraught but misunderstood. It is possible the emotionally distraught individual is eccentric and has a "past history" and may unfortunately be easily thrown into a psychiatric hospital, again based on his/her "history." Also, it is possible the person is having a side-effect to a medication, misunderstood, or an unresolved "difficult" past as were many times the cases with me. The public needs to be aware that people may possibly "fall through the cracks" as being mislabeled and once again perpetuate the steps of being wrongfully committed into a psychiatric hospital. Public awareness needs to be made aware of how easily someone can be misunderstood then labeled with a diagnosis whom the individual that's declared "mentally ill" doesn't agree with. My diagnosis of being labeled as a paranoid schizophrenic doesn't directly bother me, because the diagnosis doesn't get to the cause of my thoughts. What bothers me the most, is having done to me the aftermath of being determined a "paranoid schizophrenic" such as easily being admitted again into a psychiatric hospital due to stigma painting a picture that I "require hospitalization."

I've always been a "go getter" and have changed things for the better. In addition, I look for ways to make what is wrong – right. I'm positive by nature and never depressed but close to being depressed while on certain psychotropic medications. In a sense I have three negative things to go up against. First, is the system of how a person becomes committed into a psychiatric hospital. Second, is the stigma of being thought of as "mentally ill." Third, is making attempts to be better understood by friends and family through more appropriate socialization which means better communication of all those involved at home. Conversely, friends and family need to make efforts to understand me.

I believe many things will change in psychiatry within the next decade. I also believe a person that has a true mental health condition needs to have the symptoms for over six months before being diagnosed a certain mental health diagnosis and not one day as was in my case when first diagnosed leading to subsequent wrongful inpatient psychiatric hospitalizations.

The term "mentally ill" should be used with caution, because it refers to someone with a disease. Psychiatry has no basis of showing someone scientifically being "chemically imbalanced" – there are no blood tests. A person is better to be described as having emotional trauma. Psychiatry should focus on one's spirit and emotions and not thought of as a disease of the brain, because disease leads to wrongful connotations of treating "mental illness" with medicine as opposed to psychosocially.

Involuntary commitments into psychiatric hospitals should be more scrutinized, because the abusive tendencies of being committed when not necessary leaves an individual in family, professional, and social disarray. Unless, you lose your Rights as a person being committed into a psychiatric hospital or other confinement, it's difficult to fathom what it's like without your ability to use your phone, watch television in your own home, or be forced into treatment etc. Psychiatry must change a system that merely requires a doctor to check a box which will take an already vulnerable person's Rights away. It's difficult to at first comprehend how checking a box by a doctor can be so detrimental, but each time my Rights were taken away by the doctor trying to error on "being safe." What about my Rights as a person?

Chapter Three

Pacifying "Them"

The petition process may be the first legal document in committing someone into a psychiatric hospital, however as discussed before – it's often times based out of the petitioners and the medical society being "paranoid." I believe that each and every time I was petitioned, it was done because the petitioner didn't take the time to find resolve with me and felt they felt "paranoid" of what was happening. How do I know? Because, I lived through the process of being misunderstood, not finding resolve and having people with "paranoid" thoughts of what "might" happen. In fact, I'm forced to take medicine in efforts to pacify those around me even though I've taken the lowest dose possible and "acted" well. Unfortunately, I found that many people believe psychiatry as opposed to the patient - and would rather force someone into taking medicine even though it causes anguish, stress, and duress on the patient as was the case in myself for the past 30 years! Most recently, I'll be talking with the supervisor of the mental health department here in town to continue talk therapy after the court order expires in efforts individuals around me will understand that I will not be on medicine after the order and that talk therapy will be my "therapy" in addition to more thoughtful socialization. In addition, appropriate socialization is just as important, if not even more important than just talk therapy with a therapist. Good communication which influences my positive attributes and with optimism is the best form of therapy of which I truly believe.

I feel as though I have to currently take medicine until people are more comfortable with the thought I'm not taking medicine in order to pacify them. The thought that I must take medicine to pacify those around me isn't fair to me but it's a circumstance I'm willing to sacrifice temporarily until "they" are more comfortable with who I am.

It will be comforting to the naysayers in knowing that I've finally found resolve in my past with expressions such as writing this book in helping, and will most likely not have any more "delusions" or hallucinations because I'm finally finding closure.

Chapter Four

Educating Police Officers

Police officers are often times called to the scene of an incident to make peace of a situation or proceed with further legal ramifications. However, a specialized unit such as a rapid response mental health unit with the training done with the involvement of social work and mental health professionals trained to empathize and deescalate a situational condition will be involved first with the troubled mental health condition person. A police officer is educated in the legalities of making an arrest. How well rehearsed are officers in psychological aspects or disputes?

An educated police officer that is also empathetic of mental health patients will be more knowledgeable and have more confidence in determining, if an individual requires a mental health rapid response unit.

The police officer should ask pertinent questions to determine if the person requires the use of a Soteria house. For instance, in my case, if the police officer would have asked me questions he/she would have easily concluded that I was merely expressing my personal freedom of free speech and not required hospitalization, but perhaps just a therapist/Psychologist to talk to or a stay in a Soteria house for a brief period of time. I could certainly think clearly it may be thought of as eccentric in me distributing flyers, but I was not a threat to myself, anyone else, and I could certainly take care of myself. If things were different, the officer could have encouraged me to visit a Soteria House. I certainly would have been fine in visiting a Soteria House and may have even been cured my condition. The police officer and psychiatry in general, should be more aware of community resources in helping an individual as a sort of outpatient treatment. In addition, community resources such as drop-in shelters should be aware to the officers in case during an alleged mental health condition incident. I may have been more communicative and focused on other things than my flyers and protest, if I were taken to a place where I could socialize such as a Soteria house. Instead, the petition once again led to a one way road to being wrongfully hospitalized. There needs to be more options available to the police and psychiatry in having a person rest as a place not requiring involuntary commitment in a psychiatric hospital. In addition to Soteria houses, there may be area churches, veteran assemblies etc. in finding a refuge for the alleged "mentally ill" individual.

Once again, however it goes to show society lives in fear, stigma and social prejudices when it involves people with a "history of mental illness." I was committed each time but never lost sight of who I truly was at all times – a caring, knowledgeable person that was misunderstood and had broken relationships in communicating with friends and family. Something I knew even more about myself is that I enjoyed learning and reading.

Education is apparent in many fields and require it to maintain work. As a Nurse I'm required to complete certified course work within every two years. One of these requirements involves pain assessments plus a catalog of other medical subjects. The course work strengthens my understanding of taking care of patients and creates a more empathetic care of people in general. Police officers would also gain more empathy towards mental health patients, if they are required to devote part of their required learning towards mental health and learning of community resources that may be used in helping a person with a mental health condition.

Education is important for gaining police officer confidence in making decisions to pursue possible helping individuals with a mental health condition. The officers may gain the additional knowledge of assessing an alleged mentally ill/emotionally distraught individual by learning more about how places like Soteria houses help people with a mental heal condition. In addition, police officers need to be familiar with community services available to individuals that may require psychological or shelter resources. Patients that are "frequent flyers" should have with them a reference card also known as "crisis cards." The crisis cards are used as reference to preferred treatment of various Soteria houses, therapists, Psychologists, and medication (if chosen by the mental health patient before eventually being weaned off of them).

Police officers are our force in society, but they must gain experience in behavioral/psychological aspects as nurses are required to fulfill clinical hours on a psychiatric unit and eventually learn more about Soteria houses as a new movement in treating/curing people of a mental health condition.

Education and clinical experience will also create a more empathetic police officer that is more apt to ask the right questions and inspire a more peaceful resolution to circumstances. Police officers make decisions that influence a person's lifetime and should be educated with experience in how to perceive individuals with an emotional circumstance "mental illness." A police officer that transported me to an inpatient psychiatric hospital from a pick-up order would have easily come to the conclusion that I merely needed guidance in how I made my point across. The officer may have directed me to also have either talked to a newspaper editor or perhaps even a therapist and or Psychologist in expressing my thoughts and concerns.

Soteria houses are the least restrictive and most effective way in helping someone with a mental health condition. An on-call therapist, Psychologist or visit at a Soteria house and better communication with family and friends is all I ever needed concerning "helping" my mental health condition. I know that I certainly didn't need a 30 day stay in a psychiatric hospital forcing me to take medication as was the case many times as evident from being misunderstood due to lack of communication and empathy by the petitioner and being pushed through the medical model of psychiatry. If medication is prescribed, it should be with the premise that the mental health condition person be weaned off of them. In essence, writing this book has been a good stress reliever and all that I truly needed from the beginning which was to be heard, justice to be served in addition to a court case settlement to relieve my anguish etc. and teach/abolish psychiatry as we know it.

Education creates empathy and understanding. A beautiful result to more educated police officers would be a more satisfied society with a willingness to contribute to the profession of legal justice. Police officers would be revered by both society and at each individual encounter, if they were more educated with emotionally distraught individuals and learned the benefits of Soteria houses. Society in general would be much "happier" knowing police officers are held to a higher level of education and understanding. I believe police officers themselves will appreciate a more autonomous role compared to being a taxi like service for pick-up order to the hospital as is currently in place.

I have found through the years of being a registered nurse for nearly 14 years, licensed practical nurse for 2 years, mental health worker for 2 years and direct care worker for 4 years is that I appreciated learning more. Learning more generally gains autonomy, breaks down prejudices and frees the enslaved ways of thinking. I believe police officers will deep down inside themselves appreciate the contribution of being more empathetic and the importance of Soteria houses. Unfortunately, for me and close family and friends being "evaluated" wrongfully always ended up with me going through the one way channel and led to another treacherous, stressful, full of anguish and separation from family and friends inpatient psychiatric hospitalization.

The path between petition order and psychiatric hospitalization needs to be broken, because it is much too easy for people like me with a "history" to once again be needlessly admitted into a psychiatric hospital. I play the scenario in my head each day when I think of how easily the trip was from pick-up order to psychiatric hospitalization. I believe educating police officers is a win-win situation for the police officers, medical systems and community. Individuals like me - that fall through the cracks of being eccentric at times when trying to make resolve, and/or had side-effects to psychotropic medications which made them hallucinate and be "delusional" will also benefit in preventing an unnecessary psychiatric hospital admission and most certainly encourage the appreciation and use of a Soteria house, Psychologist or therapist.

Chapter Five

Empathy

Empathy is a strong concept that unfortunately not many people practice in their day to day living and interactions with other people. The concept of being able to put your place in the shoes of another person is the art of empathy. Understanding other people's feelings and thoughts as seen from that person's perspective is also the art of empathy. Empathy needs to be very important in psychiatry both as a professional and as a person making a petition against an alleged "mentally ill" individual to help distinguish the cause of a person's behavior. Psychotherapy by psychiatrists is a lost art unfortunately, in today's mental health arena. The practice of empathy should be a daily activity for all psychiatrists. Otherwise, psychiatrists would be equivalent to drug pushers and not caring of their patient's emotions and true feelings.

I believe having empathy must be a priority in the psychiatric profession, because when we lose sight of how the patient is truly feeling is when we lose sight of the patient. It is unfortunate that all my experiences resulted in medication taking as opposed to truly exploring my thoughts and feelings by a psychiatrist or even the petitioner, family, and friends. Empathy is vitally important and an art that needs to find its way back to psychiatry and every-day living.

Talking to an alleged "mentally ill" individual is perhaps the only therapy in addition to better communication and appropriate socialization that is needed for the alleged "mentally ill" individual to break free from their delusion, psychosis or even hallucination. Talk therapy with a therapist/Psychologist is important, however good communication and understanding by family and friends is the most important. In addition, being patient by both the petitioner and alleged "mentally ill" individual is important, because after all the alleged "mentally ill" individual has had their emotions tumultuously burdened for perhaps many years and requires patience and understanding in finding resolve with their troubled past. The possible petitioner requires patience and good communication with the alleged "mentally ill individual" and they will soon discover as was evident in my case that their walls of fear of the alleged "mentally ill" individual will break down and once again understand the person, but must be given the chance. Once understanding of the alleged "mentally ill" individual is present through better communication, then people will notice that inpatient psychiatric hospitalization is not required.

Professionals may sympathize with what the patient experienced but until the patient's true feelings are expressed will they begin to heal. Its been nearly 30 years that I've tried to be heard and have my feelings expressed. My time in the psychiatric arena shouldn't be consumed with other therapies other than "talk therapy" with Psychologists or therapists and good communication and socialization with friends and family. Empathy is an important concept and shouldn't be taken lightly. After all, understanding the other person is understanding yourself and the benefits of psychotherapy and in essence what psychiatry should achieve.

The art of empathy is a beautiful thing which many times breaks down walls of misunderstanding and anger. Empathy can help pacify a situation and encourage resolve. Mental health, legal authorities, friends, and family need to develop good empathetic communication to achieve more understanding and less hostility.

A person that has empathy understands the patient and doesn't merely with force coerce the patient into following a drug regimen. Empathy relieves tension and makes for an easy environment. The patient feels at ease and begins to break down the walls between individuals when communicating. It is important for the patient to be heard and not feel as if they are a robot like object only taking medications to pacify an oppressive psychiatric system or misunderstanding friends and family.

Visiting a psychiatrist to me is dehumanizing because my thoughts are not explored and yet I'm forced to take medicine. The result of my thoughts not being explored leaves me feeling empty inside like a shell. Psychiatrists today lack the essential work quality of empathy. How do psychiatrists know what the patient is thinking if the psychiatrists don't explore their patient's thoughts? Psychiatrists will gain favor of their patients and prevent any relapse, if they better understand their patients. It seems trivial, however psychiatrists don't practice empathy during their encounters with their patients.

I'm still astonished and have distaste for psychiatry after all the years of mental abuse I endured by mental health professionals especially psychiatrists, because they lack empathy. I'm convinced that if I were to have sit down with my mental health professionals, psychiatrists, and petitioner during my encounters in psychiatric evaluations, then I wouldn't still be in the psychiatric system. To be empathetic one must first ask questions but because psychiatrists don't ask pertinent questions that evoke feelings and current thoughts during their visit with their patient, empathy is lost. I encourage wholeheartedly every mental health professional, family and friends that question the concerned alleged "mentally ill" individual to ask them questions and find out what they are truly feeling, and thinking because it takes time to reverse the distraught emotions which scarred the alleged "mentally ill" individual. Resolving a distraught past through talk therapy with a Psychologist, therapist, and appropriate socialization with family friends through good communication makes for the healthiest recovery.

Empathy in day to day living involves understanding and knowing other people's character. The character of another person involves knowing their emotional and physical strengths and weaknesses. In addition, understanding the character of other people creates for a sense of calm and reduces apprehension and anxiety.

Chapter Six

Therapies

Many different therapies exist in treating a mental health patient. The pharmaceutical companies very much push medicine as the mainstay for treating individuals with a mental health condition. I began taking first generation psychotropic medications since I was first involuntarily hospitalized, but now take the second generation –as forced for both by court orders. I witnessed terrible side-effects from both the first and second generation medications. For instance, Haldol made me very uncomfortable like a zombie robot that drooled, hallucinated, and was even delusional. The list of medications and side-effects go on and on. A good Psychologist, therapist, being understood by family and friends is more important to me than any psychotropic medications.

I have had many therapists in my involvement with the mental health system. A good Psychologist or therapist is like a friend that explores life and asks the right questions in a manner that is not pushing medicine. The tone of voice and how they ask questions or make comments is important in building a friend-like acquaintance. A good therapist is one that you can share your thoughts with and discuss matters that are closest to the heart. If you anticipate having a good time and explore at times controversial topics during the meeting, then that is a Psychologist/therapist worth talking to. What I refer to as "talk therapy" helps me the most, because it is free from the medical model of psychiatry which pushes me through psychiatry with influence of the pharmaceutical industry. The form of therapy I favor the most – "talk therapy" is patient centered and allows me to be understood expressing my true thoughts, not what psychiatrists mention to keep me in the psychiatric system.

Other therapies exist such as electroshock but they have been noted as having terrible side-effects as memory loss and confusion.

People are speaking out against various psychiatric medications and therapies such as electroshock, also in protest to their Rights being taken away and involuntarily forced treatments.

Any therapy without consent such as during an involuntary admission takes the Rights away from the patient of which is now a victim due to the oppressive psychiatric system. How would you like to be involuntarily committed and be forced to take medications? I think we all know the answer to that rhetorical question. That is why I believe the least invasive treatment is the most righteous and effective. Psychiatry involves subjective diagnoses, because there are no blood tests to determine brain chemical imbalances or inflammation etc. Many of the medications prescribed by psychiatrists involve brain chemicals which through trial and error determine, if they are right for the individual. The trial and error is evident how the person behaves on the medication, but ultimately the decision to have medication should be the patient's and not forced into taking medication. If the person is taking medication, then the individual should also see a Psychologist/ therapist to talk about their psychosocial issues to better understand their psyche or "spirit." Psyche literally translated from the Greek language means – "spirit/soul. I believe, modern psychiatry needs to re-visit the person as having an ailing, or overly-strong spirit/soul that may be misunderstood. Psychiatrists should also, begin weaning patients off psychotropic medications from the day medication is started due to the deleterious long term possible side-effects of psychotropic medications. If medicine is started, they should be given on the premise for a person to develop effective coping strategies then slowly weaned off them. Psychiatry should focus more on the psyche or spirit/soul of an individual and not concentrate on the brain as having a "disease." There are no scientific tests to show brain chemical imbalances or even the newest theory of inflammation in the brain, but social interactions often times transpire the worst case environment for the distraught/alleged "mentally ill" individual. Therefore, talk therapy as with a Psychologist/therapist or personal communication with family and friends will allow for the patient to better understand the psychosocial aspect of behavior – a true manifestation of the brain.

There exists organizations within the U.S. for people that have witnessed harm while being in the psychiatric arena as a patient. Organizations specific to mental health believe in being psychiatric survivors. They know and have witnessed people harmed by psychiatry either emotionally with a label they know not to be true, or medications and procedures with terrible often permanent side-effects. A psychiatric survivor is a person that was most often involuntarily taking medications or other forms of therapy and are now free from psychiatry living - healthy and productive lives.

I Thank GOD for organizations for psychiatric survivors to describe their stories, and seek help or at least make friends and find strength in numbers that inspire living free from forced treatments. Let's face it, being forced to be confined in a mental hospital then to take medications against their will takes away Rights and is a form of mental rape causing the alleged "mentally ill" person: grief, anguish, stress, and duress. A rape that takes away a person's thinking, beliefs, and present lifestyle. In addition, what else can be said about the friends and family that are left to fend for themselves when a person is involuntarily taken away into a psychiatric hospital?

I live life as much I can to the fullest every day. I live, however knowing that I must take my medication through a court order which I now have begrudgingly agreed to be injected by a nurse every month as opposed to oral medication which the doctor hasn't talked about as an option. I take my medication against my will, but I still find in myself to be happy, because I haven't lost sight of who I truly am. I thank GOD for my sense of humor, kindness, knowledge, empathy, and thankfulness in helping people especially as a professional Registered Nurse. As I mentioned earlier, I would be a successful Nurse Practitioner now, if I hadn't started to distribute flyers, dealt with non-empathetic systems such as psychiatry, then "let go" from my graduate nursing program.

Therapy can be anything that makes us feel good, and reflect on who we are. Activities such as gardening, riding my bike, walking my dog, drawing and of course being with my children, close family and friends makes me happy. I truly find happiness, but in general am a happy guy to begin with. It doesn't take much to make me happy. Perhaps, what makes me the happiest is knowing that I have helped someone live a better more full holistic life. It isn't too often when people hear or read stories of individuals expressing how "happy" they are, but I believe helps ignite more feelings of other people in thinking positively of their everyday life situations.

My contributions in helping my parents can't be bought with all the money in the world. I make time in helping my mother (my father passed away in hospice at the age of 86 years old) throughout the day, and take pride of her good health. I put my 100% in being the best at what I do. No one can take away all the lives I saved while working in an acute care hospital as a charge or floor nurse. I will say that, if all people seen my accomplishments, I would never have been committed into a psychiatric hospital. Being successful at helping people is in itself therapy for me.

I care of my "diagnosis" but don't let my thoughts of how I'm perceived bother me, because I know who I am and don't let superficial prejudices bother me. I will always fight for the person I know I am and always was. It's a crying shame how backwards and dark being on the wrong side of psychiatry truly is, as I've personally witnessed. Psychiatry needs to be aware that something might be wrong with the system when people fight in clearing themselves from their psychiatric "therapies." I believe doctors truly need to make an appointment with the patient and ask pertinent questions that may rule out a diagnosis and not automatically label a person. Many factors including environmental are modifiable and should be used as a method in ruling out any possible diagnosis. Making a diagnosis in psychiatry should involve analysis of an individual's psyche as well as modifiable and social factors.

Love to me is the best therapy. As long as I can love someone, share kindness, and be understood with a resolved past – these are truly the most important therapies. Sharing good times as at a dinner or around a fire place with my significant other is also a form of love that I cherish. I thank GOD for adults that I can share life's experiences and not expect a favor in return. Life could be better, but with love there isn't much that could even come close to making me sad. I believe there are three forms of love. There is love for being with family, friends, and self. There is also love in doing something that a person truly enjoys and there is love in a significant other. Realizing all the different forms of love and having harmony with life truly makes for a fulfilling day of happiness.

The outcome to the truest form of therapy is having peace with yourself. I can honestly say that I'm happy, but could be happier knowing my children will always be with me and I eventually find resolve with my past as through expressing myself as in doing things like writing this book. I'm happy with myself and have a good conscience in helping those around me. I ask those that are reading my book to find it within yourself to have a greater conscience and make yourself happy by helping others and above all - find love and live with harmony. A life without love and harmony within its environment is lost and cold.

The travesty lies in the personal belief that all I needed was a good Psychologist or therapist to talk to and have good communication with family and friends in being understood and dealing with medication side-effects which were even forced onto me. Instead, I was left with publicly displaying my frustrations with flyers and hoped I would be understood. I have had good Psychologists and therapists in the past where I have mentioned many pertinent things in life of which I could cope with, but now it's time to focus on the secret I've kept for 30 years – the unprofessional remark made by my first psychiatrist and incidence at company "Y." That psychiatrist – Dr."X," has no idea how much he messed up my life! For years I displayed my mentions in the form of flyers, taken medications I felt didn't need, and even given a label of being a "paranoid schizophrenic" which set me up to be once again "diagnosed" and misunderstood as part of the psychiatric realm and still in the system 30 years later.

The next session I have with my Psychologist/therapist will no longer keep Dr. "X" a secret. I will talk to my therapist about a topic that truly needs mention. I will tell her what Dr. "X" had said, and that will be a topic we can truly talk about. Dr. "X" is probably nearly 70-80 years old now as I'm not sure where he is. I've tried finding him before my experiences with the internet and have asked my case manager to find more information about him. At the very least it will be a sense of closure in a way to see his picture again. I will never forget what he said and how I reacted by calmly going back to my room and throwing a chair at my inpatient psychiatric hospital room's window to make a point of how unprofessional his comment was by myself making a commotion. I wasn't paranoid and didn't necessarily believe what he had said, but still am having a difficult time forgiving his words. I eventually will forgive and forget, when I have reached closure and resolve. Once again, writing and being understood is a good form of both – closure and resolve. Perhaps, I can now get on with the rest of my life as more people are understanding me by listening to what I have to say and reading my book, but first I still need to talk with a Psychologist/ therapist about the past 30 years of my life. The past 30 years of my life have been the most misunderstood and left in turmoil. It is unfortunate that I've been trying to let my concerns known while a "patient" in psychiatry, but believe I will have better recourse in standing up for the real me by voicing and writing how difficult the past 30 years of my life have been. Expressing my feelings and thoughts is a way of relieving my stress by being understood.

Therapy involves mentioning something that is relevant and working on issues to help find peace within the soul. Something needs to be said regarding my frustrations while hospitalized and involuntary confinement in the various multiple psychiatric units. I have called and written the Rights advisor and even state authorities of why I didn't need to be in a psychiatric unit. I notified Rights advisors nearly every day that I was hospitalized explaining I was confined for no real psychiatric reason and got no positive response. I have let many people know of my anguish, stress, and duress I personally went through while a psychiatric patient by psychiatry but no one seems to understand or shows to care of my negative experiences in the mental health system until now. Once again, I'm left with the feeling that nothing is being done about my concerns until I believe more people understand me and my tumultuous time in the field of psychiatry as a patient – until now. Expressing myself through words is a justifiable means of gaining some relief and think that I may actually be heard.

Each hospitalization was met with me writing furiously to the Rights advisor how I didn't need to be in the psychiatric hospital. This book is truly a tool that gets my point across and will help to mend my spirit/soul and bring light to the reasons of why I have behaved the way I have over the past years – in finding resolve for my distraught past. In addition, it has not been fully recognized that my spirit/soul was hurt when treated by therapies such as forced medication and wrongful psychiatric ward lock ups, which I obviously didn't approve of.

Where do I begin with what I'd like to tell Dr. "X?" If it weren't for my fight for justice and resolve I would easily be practicing as a Family Nurse Practitioner in Psychiatry and maybe even changed how psychiatry practices health, but this book and being better understood may help change Psychiatry and better make me more understood. I held honors in both undergraduate and graduate school. In addition, I have two Bachelor's degrees, one in Nursing and the other in Biology. I'm proud of myself and believe GOD put me through difficult times and being misunderstood to triumph and be an inspiration to other people.

Writing this book made me wonder what I would be doing after I graduated as a Family Nurse Practitioner. I thought to myself that I would probably have gone further in my education and completed a post graduate degree in efforts to have a dual degree as a psychotherapist. Either way I hope to influence psychiatry, mental health field, family and friends to listen to their patients and family members, encourage better communication/socialization, rule out mental health diagnoses, consider environmental, and modifiable factors as to the reason for someone acting strangely or bazaar, and realize the time frame of the person's symptoms.

I recently discovered a form of treatment involving staff that are not necessarily medical staff in what is called a Soteria house. A Soteria house was first introduced by a psychiatrist named Loren Mosher in the 60's during deinstitutionalization of psychiatric patients. The Soteria house uses staff with creative empathy and understanding in "treating" their patients. Medication is an option not encouraged but close staff interactions and arts/crafts as well as other hobbies are a part of daily living at the house. The important virtues of respect and care is expressed at the Soteria house and "patients" are free to enter and leave whenever they choose. The concept of the Soteria house is a beautiful notion and certainly a prospective option for me instead of involuntary inpatient psychiatric hospitalization – if I were ever given the choice from another wrongful petition then psychiatrically "evaluated" for placement.

The pharmaceutical industry, unfortunately infiltrated how mental health patients were treated and psychiatrists began prescribing psychotropics. Unfortunately, patients were negatively affected by the prescriptive phase of psychiatry, because what the patients were truly thinking was lost due to psychiatrists prescribing meds – losing patient/staff dialogue and understanding.

Chapter Seven

Psychosocial vs. Illness/Disease Models of Mental Health

Shouldn't psychiatry be more concerned with helping the individual and not about the fear of what may happen if a person isn't taking their court ordered prescribed medications? What happened to psychiatry's help of the patient? Psychiatry needs to move away from the "illness" and "disease" model of diagnosing patients and focus more on the psychosocial aspects of which may influence a person's behavior and delve into their psyche or spirit/soul of who they are. Psychiatrists must also include modifiable factors such as: lack of resolve, environmental, food allergies, medications, sleep deprivation, malnutrition, and hypothermia as contributing to a person's mental health condition. I further believe, that if a person has symptoms of being mentally ill/emotionally distraught but are attributed to modifiable factors then that patient shouldn't have a declared diagnosis such as schizophrenia but rather an acute circumstantial incident resulting from a modifiable factor.

Even the healthiest of individuals may hallucinate, if they have inadequate sleep, allergies to food/medicine, or unresolved situations. For instance, books have been written describing even the healthiest of men - Navy Seals hallucinating and being delusional during their training due to inadequate sleep and stress. A psychiatrist should devote most of his/her assessments exploring the non-organic - natural and environmental factors which may contribute to psychiatric conditions before concluding a diagnosis. A medical diagnosis is difficult to expunge from one's personal records, because I believe each medical doctor builds on the reference of previous doctor's opinions and an entire lifetime of a patient could be innocently lost in a misdiagnosis or harmful treatment. Making a psychiatric diagnosis should be done while ruling out possible environmental-modifiable factors. A diagnosis should also be scrutinized by each newly seen psychiatrist and not based on patient "history" or past doctors.

A diagnosis in mental health should be determined with patient presiding symptoms that last over six months. I felt as though my first diagnosis which occurred in 1990 with symptoms that lasted one day, was used as a diagnosis each time during hospitalization. Doctors need to be held accountable to ruling out environmental factors before determining a true "schizophrenic" or manic depressive etc. The DSM – medical book in creating diagnosis shouldn't focus on diagnosis but instead the cause of the patient's distraught emotions etc. Doctors must consider the condition not only as the patient was described as being by bystanders or witnesses, because that is merely hearsay and mostly inaccurate. Thoughtfully asking appropriate questions may break the chain of previous misdiagnosis or determine better treatment opportunities. Personal experience with psychiatric visits were with the doctor asking me what happened to get me hospitalized. What about my current beliefs? What happened that got me hospitalized was many times based on hearsay and "old news." Psychiatrists need to focus on where the patient is now in their thinking not necessarily on old interviews or petitions even being a day old.

Modifiable factors such as side-effects from psychotropic medications played a role in me being "delusional" and even hallucinatory. Many of my involuntary psychiatric visits were protests to a label of being a paranoid schizophrenic which I objected to being mislabeled, because I believe it's not true as was based on hearsay and/or even malice, and unresolved distraught past. After all, I have a medical background and know what I've witnessed in my lifetime. In addition, I also can view how my life could have been misunderstood, given how I must have "appeared" to a person or medical professional that didn't ask me pertinent questions in relation to my presiding condition. Without appropriate questioning what my beliefs were, I can understand how my life was misunderstood for 30 years by a system that was not empathetic but oppressive.

In retrospect, I may have been anxious briefly in my life - 30 years ago while living in the city of Detroit, but that was on very little to no sleep, poor eating habits and difficult living conditions. In addition, I no longer take first generation psychotropic medications which made me have side-effects of me hallucinating and being delusional. I'm a full-time working Registered Nurse. I have accomplished many things in life including raising my son, visiting/being with my daughter, working full time as a Registered Nurse, caretaker of my parents and two Bachelor degrees – one in Nursing and the other in Biology. I'm also a respectable citizen and father figure.

The mental health condition/disease model of psychiatry is presently being used which grossly undermines the environmental aspects of mental health. The term delusion may not be appropriate and is often times used erroneously even by doctors making a misdiagnosis, if they don't ask the appropriate questions. Only a very small percentage of the population have true delusions and hallucinations that are not related to modifiable factors. My personal experiences with psychiatrists haven't explored my thoughts of what I did or even question what my true beliefs were or currently are. Psychiatrists have quickly judged and came to the conclusion that I was delusional in thinking company "Y" owed me money in an "out of court case settlement," but failed to ask me the point of my settlement.

The mental health condition/disease model of psychiatry determines the person to be mentally ill as if they have diabetes etc., but the brain is more flexible and malleable than any medical definition. The brain is ever changing with some good days and some bad. How is it that the doctor or anyone else can be with the patient 24/7 to determine what the person actually believes or is living a delusion? The doctor should perceive the patient's thoughts of how they feel as being the true definition of how they are. Psychiatry is not like other fields which have clinical tests to prove a medical condition. For instance, the field of psychiatry can't prove anyone has a chemical imbalance showing a certain neurotransmitter needs to be corrected. The chemical disease model is even being refuted by many professionals as being erroneous.

A diagnosis in mental health should be scrutinized by each psychiatrist during each encounter. The issue lies with how difficult it is to seek and obtain retributions. Receiving retributions or seeking justice to what Dr."X" said 30 years ago shouldn't be this difficult. I did let some people know about Dr. "X"'s unprofessional remarks nearly 30 years ago but my voice fell on deaf ears. A sort of "big brother" system over psychiatrists needs to be put in place. At the very least, the Rights advisors we have now should be more in tuned with properly doing their job. I have been wrongfully involuntarily committed into a psychiatric hospital many different times. How many times have I been contacted outside of the hospital as any follow up to what may have been done regarding my complaints? The answer is not one time did I receive a follow up phone call out of concern of my Rights or treatment!

The Rights advisor should have it to be their job in meeting with the person making the Right's complaint. A face to face meeting is important to gain empathy and ask the person complaining of their Rights – questions. Follow up after the hospital stay should also be carried out by the Rights advisor to determine if any additional action needs to be taken against the medical professional. A truly dedicated Rights advisor will investigate the person's complaint and make a follow-up of any evidence they discovered concerning the individual's complaint. If no follow ups are done by the Rights advisor, then how can we be sure the complainant was being heard? I have no reason to believe anything was done by the Rights advisor with regards to all my complaints even from 30 years ago! Patients need some kind of reassurance that they are being heard and that their concerns are cared for in solving. The more empathetic and understanding the Rights advisor the more sincere they will be in answering the complainants concerns.

Psychiatry should be seen as a field that deals with human emotions and spirit/soul. Psychotherapy delves into the patient's psyche and mentions emotions as a humanistic quality and not a diseased state. Very few individuals have non-modifiable factors contributing to their illness. In addition, a person with a mental health diagnosis shouldn't be casted aside as always having that diagnosis, because people can heal through appropriate socializations and expressions of thoughts etc.

Changes to the disease model need to focus less on the brain requiring medication for its remedy, but on healing the soul and psychology of the patient through better communication with family and friends and talk therapy with a therapist. If the disease model is kept in its form, then psychiatry will too easily fall in the trap of only prescribing medications or other forms not delving into the psyche of the individual as its main treatment options. I believe, psychiatrists prescribe psychotropic medications in efforts to see many patients a day in the least amount of time all while billing insurance for each patient encounter. It is also easier for psychiatrists to follow up with patients even in large numbers if medications are prescribed as opposed to the most gainful form of therapy – talk therapy. Psyche comes from the Greek word meaning doctor of the spirit/soul. I believe the ancient Greeks were accurate in focusing on the spirit of psychiatry and looking into the patient's heart and soul. After all, if the spirit/soul is not healed then often times the body will seem as though something is wrong or at the very least like there is an insult similar to war.

Chapter Eight

Visiting the Psychiatrist

Visits to the psychiatrist should focus not just on the actions of the patient which got them hospitalized, or even often times the false petition remarks and being misunderstood, but their true current thoughts and beliefs. A good psychiatrist doesn't react quickly in concluding a medical diagnosis. Instead, a psychiatrist should ask pertinent questions such as, what did he, or she mean by this and currently believe? In my most recent inpatient involuntary psychiatric hospitalizations, I distributed flyers as a last resort because my concerns fell on deaf ears for years. A truly thorough exam would delve into the psyche of the patient and even develop empathy and knowledge of their background, at home experiences, and environment. Unfortunately, medications have been prevalent with each psychiatric encounter I've had. I would be more open to treatment, if talk therapy was the sole intervention. In addition, family and friends should be included in efforts to promote good communication and socialization which would prevent another misunderstanding. I believe I should have the final say of what I ingest or happens to me with regards to the type of treatment involved with psychiatry. I should have the Right to refuse medication but stay with talk therapy. I have found with all my years of being a mental health patient that psychiatry is coercive and oppressive in making the patient take medication. In addition, psychiatry has been mentally abusive towards me because they assumed I didn't know what's right for myself and must be under the coercive demand of the psychiatrist and therapist. In addition, I believe psychiatry is oppressive in that there is no way for the patient to prove the psychiatrist or therapist is wrong due to the psychiatric system placing judgements of "poor insight" or "failure to recognize need for treatment" when the patient attempts to defend themselves from current psychiatric malpractice.

It is true that some therapists perform the function of psychotherapy, but then what is the reason for psychiatrists other than to prescribe medications? What if I don't need medications? Do I no longer need a psychiatrist? I based my comments on the experiences I've had with psychiatrists over 30 years.

A psychiatrist would be more empathetic in realizing people and patients are more than a herd of cattle as was my experience. We have feelings and thoughts that may not have been expressed to the therapist. What of our true thoughts? It is too easy to be caught in the hearsay then labeled with a misdiagnosis after a "box" was checked by the ER doctor which involuntarily commits an individual into a psychiatric unit. A psychiatrist would have more benefited me by asking personal questions and scrutinizing the diagnosis, if it were actually accurate or not. It is true that psychiatrists need a diagnosis to treat and bill insurance, but they must also consider people shouldn't be labeled as having the disease/emotional trauma or diagnosis forever. People and circumstances change. These changes and circumstances may inevitably change a psychiatrist's opinion of a person and an empathic psychiatrist may even question the diagnosis. Let's not forget that psychiatry comes from the Greek word – spirit/soul doctor, it is felt that psychiatry has lost its roots when they started treating patients with medicine and lacked insight and empathy for their patients by not asking pertinent personal questions. We must not forget that a person's spirit/soul may be hurt of which understanding their emotions and thoughts are important in understanding the patient.

What if I had a psychiatrist analyzing my thoughts – why I dispersed flyers? They would have gotten to the point of what truly bothered me. There is no medication that can ask the appropriate question that a truly knowledgeable psychiatrist focusing on my psyche can ask, but never did in the past. Psychiatrists need to spend more time with their patients or at least give more credence and confidence in the therapists that actually communicate with the patient for more than only 10 minutes as with my personally experiences with psychiatrists. A great deal of psychiatry was lost when psychotherapy was an art of the past. When psychiatrists do prescribe medications which unfortunately was 100% of the time, then a plan to eventually come off medications should also be discussed not left to a forever requirement for meds once appropriate coping strategies are created.

Coping strategies can be developed during recovery time with or without psychotropic medications. The mind is not always in a "mentally ill"/emotionally distraught state or have a wounded spirit/soul. So many factors can give the appearance of delusion or schizophrenia etc. As I mentioned before, the symptoms should persist for at least six months not merely one day as in my case. I can understand a shorter diagnosis period of a few weeks for severely mental health patients but the patient's psyche needs to be explored. Ruling out modifiable factors should also be explored and not automatically assumed the person is naturally sick and in a "mentally ill"/emotionally distraught state for the rest of their lives.

Chapter Nine

Influences of Pharmaceutical Companies on Psychiatry

Psychiatrists see many patients a day made possible by "adjusting" their medicine. It seems as though the main reason psychiatrists see patients – as was true in my personal experiences was for medication adjustments based on forced drugging through court orders. Pharmaceutical companies visit doctor's offices to display their products while often times providing the office with lunch or snacks. Unfortunately, doctors focus their visits with patients less on psychosocial aspects, environmental, and not necessarily the patient's circumstances as was my personal experiences when being "treated." Unfortunately, the mental illness and disease model are prevalent in today's world of psychiatry. Also, unfortunately - medication is the main treatment currently for the "mental illness" and "disease" model. Since the visit with the psychiatrist mostly focuses on medications, when will the patient come off the medication assuming they don't want to be on them for the rest of their life?

There needs to be more psychosocial questioning by the psychiatrists when visited by patients. Otherwise, the patient will be indefinitely taking medication and hazards of coming off medication without a psychiatrist adjusting the dosage to tapering amounts. Psychotropic medications must be tapered when coming off to prevent side-effects from occurring or their mental health condition will worsen. Side-effects to psychotropic medications are many times the reason for initially being placed on medicine, as was evident with me. Some psychotropic medication side-effects are delusions and hallucinations as was the case for me.

Generic brand medications are seldom apparent because it seems as though new medications are developed every year. The cost of brand name psychotropic medications are astronomical sometimes reaching thousands of dollars a month for one medication. I many times took advantage of free samples provided by the community of mental health, because of the high costs of the medication as I was court ordered to take medication against my will.

Patients court ordered to take medications are forced to take medications, and often times are vulnerable to side-effects because of the newer meds not disclosing full range of their effects. For instance, recent court hearings have awarded millions of dollars to male patients developing enlarged breasts after taking certain new medications. The manufacturers of these new medications didn't disclose the side-effect of gynecomastia and caused emotional harm to thousands of male patients. The psychological harm caused the manufacturer to change its chemical structure into other newer medications, but with what new side effects?

Not all medications for people are harmful. Some patients benefit from a temporary fix from medications. The more a person is taking a medication however, the greater chance of side-effects occurring. The honest and empathetic psychiatrist will begin the patient's first visit by explaining the tapering method, if he or she so chooses to come off the medication.

Each of the visits I've had with my psychiatrist hardly ended with the thought of tapering off medication. This is not to say that I needed to be on medication indefinitely. Since I've been court ordered to take medication, I must comply in doing so. Fortunately, I seem to be myself and feel like I normally did before taking the medication. Only time will tell however, because it doesn't take long for a side-effect to occur. Unfortunately, for some people a side-effect may persist for a life time. Medications should be used if a person believes they require the medication. After all, how the patient perceives himself/herself should be a priority for each doctor's visit and not a court order mandating to keep taking the medication.

The experiences I've had with psychiatrists concerning medication side-effects, was the method in testing side-effects to medications using the abnormal involuntary muscle scale (AIMS) as taught to me during my graduate school as a nurse practitioner. The AIMS test takes less than two minutes to complete and is a quick method of determining side-effects simply by having the patient stick out his/her tongue, straighten their arms and say a few phrases. The AIMS test is primarily used in determining any tardive dyskinesia also known as involuntary muscle movements due to side-effects from medications. Only, a few times was I asked before by a psychiatrist in my 30 years as a mental health patient to perform an AIMS test for medication side-effects! I urge the psychiatric profession to listen to their patients and plan for the tapering of their medication, if the patient chooses to do so. The patient is a beautiful individual and should be explored socially and psychologically not through the use of forcing medications onto them. At the very least, the psychiatrist should closely work with the therapist in asking how the patient is responding to therapy sessions and, if they have any concerns with their personal or social life.

Medications may be important for some patients, but I've always been a holistic person believing in being natural. My blood work shows all my electrolytes and thyroid hormones are normal. It is unfortunate that there are no tests to prove brain chemical balances in efforts to prove the theory wrong. I'm sure my brain chemicals are in order because I've always had my faculties except when having side-effects to psychotropic medications. Psychiatrists many times rely on what is said about the patient and papers such as petitions in basing judgement for diagnosis and possible medications. Unfortunately, psychiatrists may be influenced by other factors and people other than the patient, in making a diagnosis. Medications are a big business in the U.S. and I urge psychiatry to think of what the patient states, consider environmental, social, and modifiable aspects before determining the necessity of prescribing mind altering psychotropic medications.

I can't help but think of all the side-effects I've had over the years from scary upward curling of my eyes, gross arm involuntary muscle movements, delusions and even hallucinations from psychotropic medications. My experiences of side - effects to medications have mostly been short term. The medication I'm on has the least side-effects compared to previous court ordered medication experiences against my will. I will most likely continue with the current medication I'm taking as mandated through the court order while on court order. Newer medications which last longer are strongly considered as an option for me as it means less visits to the mental health center for the medication injections.

Medications may be important for people that actually require them and are taking them with a clear conscience and desire to do so. The pharmaceutical companies have improved their methods of purifying medications to produce fewer side effects, however assessment for side effects by the psychiatrist should be done with every visit. Time will tell if a person has a side-effect to a certain medication.

Chapter Ten

Modifiable Factors

Modern psychology has shown that our environment dramatically influences our behavior. I grew up with good and bad like everyone else, but I had an additional obstacle yet thoughtful blessing of being born and raised first generation speaking Greek at home and English in public schools. I remember translating for my parents at doctor's offices. I feel blessed knowing that I learned the Greek language effortlessly, because it was taught to me at home in every day usage and expressions. Knowing a second language opened my mind to a new culture and music. I enjoy listening to Greek music and speaking the Greek language. My mind can quickly change from understanding Greek to English and English to Greek.

I grew up in a family where we depended on each other. My family helped me by providing the necessities in life such as food, shelter, and clothing while I translated in Greek to my parents with each medical visit etc. In addition, I'm primary caretaker for both of my parents. How is it that I've been committed many different times in psychiatric hospitals – involuntarily? Part of the reason is my resolve with psychiatry and how easy it is with a person having a "history of prior psychiatric hospitalizations" involved with a system (psychiatry) and family that is not understanding or empathetic. I've discovered much of psychiatry is based on social networks – what he said - she said, and hearsay.

I've been passive in the mental health field for too long bottling in all my energy and how misunderstood I am even by my own family. I must now tell my story, however for my own sanity and show the world the "me" that enjoys being who I am and not someone other people believe me to be. The "phone game" well describes what hearsay may lead to. The "phone game" is if you were to tell a friend - say for instance about a party, the end result of how a third person may interpret what you originally said will probably be very different from what was originally said. Psychiatry can be frightening because actions of people can be misunderstood, yet the actions of court orders can force an individual into "treatment" for a long time. Psychiatry would be met with less apprehension if there was a safety net in keeping people from being court ordered into inpatient or outpatient treatment.

The environment plays a key role in how healthy a person is feeling and mental health is not different. I ask this rhetorical question, how healthy would it be to place someone in the same chaotic situation that caused grief or harm? I'm not saying I need to be removed from my environment, nearly quite the opposite. Things need to change, the mental health system needs to recognize that medications can't substitute psychotherapy and that each individual is different. Medications may work for a very small minority or not at all. I also urge the psychiatric profession to ask the patient questions. For instance, do they actually believe they are living in a delusion or were they merely trying to just make a point? In addition, does the person still believe the delusion or has it passed on its own already as was the case for many in past experiences. Also, psychiatrists need to give more credit to the patient in giving them the benefit of the doubt. In addition, therapists need to encourage family and friends to have more appropriate communication with the alleged "mentally ill" individual to better understand them in resolving a tumultuous past and finding resolve. As I mentioned earlier, there are many reasons a person may seem to have a mental health diagnosis which are controllable modifiable factors such as: a difficult past, hypothermia, malnutrition, insomnia, medication side effects, food allergies and even common medical diseases such as colds etc. All environmental factors need to be ruled out before a definitive mental health diagnosis is made. I know because my medication side-effects, and unresolved past were harmful, but I could also learn to modify my environment. Trying a different medication with fewer side-effects until coping strategies were developed may have also been a good option since I was forced to take medication through a court order.

A patient's ability to learn should also be explored as to any treatment options for the patient. A patient that learns or knows psychosocial aspects will likely benefit from talk therapy. Therefore, medication may not be the right answer. I believe that I'm intelligent and can make my own decisions regarding treatment options, where are my Rights? I'm perfectly capable and have shown with experience that I can make appointments in meeting with a therapist etc. In retrospect, I choose treatment by seeing a Psychologist or therapist which also encourages effective and appropriate social communication. It is unfortunate that I must take court ordered medication. The theme throughout my psychiatric experiences is that of trying to be heard and visiting an empathic therapist and having good communication with family and friends.

A big aspect in my situation is my freedom of treatment. My personal preference to not take medications hasn't even occurred. I was prescribed medication without even asking for my thoughts in coming off the medications or even taking them to begin with. I've had thoughts from my most recent hospitalization that psychiatry has two sides of which I'm in the dark side as opposed to the light. Psychiatry to me seems to be a field that is trying to pacify my concerns by ignoring my regards, because no one is taking the time to listen to what I'm saying, but finding some sanctity as in writing this book.

A small percentage of patients have an organic brain disease meaning there are no environmental factors or modifiable factors which can amend the mind. The vast majority of patients, however have modifiable factors which can be worked on in therapy sessions or simply a change in environment and understanding family and friends. Studies have shown twins separated at birth, with one being successful and the other one dependent upon their environment which also involved different circumstances. The circumstance of the situation makes big differences in outcome potential. For instance, the rhetorical question whom would you rather live with – a family with no financial burden or a family that can't afford electricity? Circumstance makes a big difference in creating a favorable environment for mental health. The more treacherous and difficult living condition, the more prone for mental health condition or loss of spirit to be prevalent. The less stressful living and more of being understood and good communication condition, the more prone to living without mental health condition or loss of spirit.

An empathetic psychiatrist truly understands that environment plays a key role in behavior and must ask the pertinent questions to explore any modifiable psychological factors. There is a time in everyone's life when we must release what's on our mind and make sense of our environment. A good therapist and psychiatrist recognizes the obstacles in a person's life and asks the right questions to help the patient overcome them. A good Psychologist/therapist also recognizes when to keep asking the right questions to help the patient express what is on their mind. The therapist in a sense can be considered an important part of the patient's environment, but must also learn when to let go of the patient and have the patient "fly away on their own." A good therapist also creates an environment where the patient feels safe in expressing their thoughts and explores his/her own meanings to what was said during the discussion. In addition, a good therapist will encourage good communication between family and friends to better understand the patient.

We all know the answer to, can a doctor or anyone be with a person all the time and know what the person is thinking? The answer is, of course not. Psychiatrists must in fact be diligent about environmental factors and be careful to rule out modifiable factors before making a diagnosis. Making a diagnosis without recognizing possible modifiable factors is like placing a band aid on a wound without getting to the root of the cause of the problem. I also know for a fact that Haldol made me hallucinate visual objects in addition to making me feel like a zombie that drooled and felt delusional. There are a list of side- effects I can mention with all more than six different psychotropic medications I've taken. The bad side effects to medicine were uncomfortable and the worst side-effects were unbearable such as that which I had with Prolixin. Prolixin was given to me about 18 years ago and the side effect from that injectable medication made my eyes turn towards the ceiling. The turning of my eyes was so harsh that I feared my retinas were going to snap! I nearly blindly made my way to the nurses' station in the psychiatric hospital and pleaded for the nurse to give me an anecdote to the medication. She came back with an injection of Cogentin which within a few minutes subsided the terrifying side-effect. New research has discovered that food additives have caused hallucinations in children. The different forms of modifiable environmental factors described earlier must be explored before medication is administered and a definitive diagnosis made. Symptoms lasting more than six months should be considered indicative of a mental health condition.

Many factors may actually cause the appearance of a mental health condition. We must also consider other environmental factors not yet discovered which may cause hallucinations and delusions. A very small percentage of people have a true mental health condition. Most mental health conditions can be explained and are attributed to environmental and modifiable factors. It is up to the clinician/psychiatrist to determine the cause and not automatically assume it's an organic meaning natural and prescribe medications.

A modifiable factor can be removed from the environment or added to it to mend the individual's mental health condition. For instance, as in the case of my first psychiatric admission, I could have just stayed home and thought about what the doctor had said which was unprofessional, in an attempt to make resolve. In addition, I could have made myself something nutritious to eat like a bowl of oatmeal, because I wasn't eating well at the time. Another modifiable factor I could have analyzed was the fact that I hallucinated and was delusional on certain psychotropic medication side-effects. The doctor was aware of the side- effects from the psychotropic medications and took me off them and then prescribed different medications still against my will – as I was court ordered to take medicine.

Chapter Eleven

Remedies to Modifiable Factors

Depending on the modifiable factor, each method to remedy a mental health system is individualized. For instance, the food should be removed from the person, if it is determined to cause a hallucinogenic response. One way to detect if the person has a reaction to a food is by slowly adding or eliminating one food for every week's duration and notice the patient's response. There was actually a supposition that certain food additives in potato chips caused hallucinogenic responses in people. Many of us are aware of some of the red and yellow food coloring dyes also causing psychiatric conditions such as anxiety and attention deficit disorder. Children with an inadequate diet of fish – at least two servings of fish a week have been susceptible to attention deficit disorder as described in research journals. The role of food plays an important factor in good mental health. Vegetables such as cauliflower and broccoli are determined to be good brain foods.

Insomnia which has been known to cause delusions and hallucinations in extreme cases, may be cured with methods such as yoga, warm water with honey, massages, and exercise. Exercise shouldn't be done within two hours of sleep time, because the body may still be revving up to boost for energy causing the opposite of being tired. Sometimes, good company and some time in a Jacuzzi are all that is needed to help relax for a good night's sleep. Try not to eat anything within two hours of sleep, because the energy required to break the food down may keep a person awake at night. Other people find reading a book helpful in falling asleep. Make every attempt to keep the bedroom a place for sleep. Don't play the television or eat in bed. You may find having curtains specially designed to block the light out helpful in helping to relax. Medications may certainly be helpful in helping someone fall asleep but should be used as a last resort.

Some psychotropic medications may cause a person to hallucinate, be depressed or delusional. Everyone reacts differently to psychotropic medications. There is no blood test to determine chemical imbalances so it's by trial and error how patients will react to certain psychotropic medications.

Perhaps, the most concerning modifiable factor in my situation is having resolve with past experiences. I was abused as a child mentally and physically. I won't go into detail, but I will state that the abuse I endured didn't stop from childhood. Also, my first psychiatrist as stated earlier, caused a traumatic experience in my life. Finding resolve with my first psychiatrist and the incident at company "Y" will greatly positively affect my mental health condition. I've determined however, that the incidences with the psychiatrist and company "Y" have gained resolve as best as could because more people are understanding how these two incidences negatively affected my mental health as noted through therapy and better more appropriate communication with family and friends as in writing this book and making my points in being understood and by more empathic listeners.

In addition, another distant modifiable factor is being understood better by the person petitioning an individual into a psychiatric hospital. As in my case, I was misunderstood for decades and dealt with a society and even family that found it easier for them to have me committed into a psychiatric hospital as opposed to talk with me and share my feelings.

The point here is to consider all modifiable factors as reasons to the mental health condition. Only after a psychiatrist has ruled out the modifiable factors, should natural causes diagnose a mental health condition. If this were true in my case, I wouldn't have stepped foot one time in a psychiatric hospital. It is very important for care providers such as psychiatrists to not make haste when diagnosing a patient. It is equally as important to not diagnose a patient based on previous diagnoses. Each patient encounter should be based on what's presented by the patient at that time. In addition, psychiatrists shouldn't be shy in using knowledge based on other fields of study. For instance, the psychiatrist Dr. "X" did make a threatening remark although I never truly felt threatened me and the next doctor I mentioned that to - shouldn't have assumed that I hallucinated what the doctor had said. Instead, a therapist should have been contacted and started therapy sessions and maybe even file a police report against the psychiatrist that said the threatening – unprofessional remark. In my case, never did my psychiatrists - after doctor "X," question that the doctor had threatened me. I did mention the threat made by my first psychiatrist to the second doctor and was met with a blank stare. The second psychiatrist labeled me as being a "paranoid schizophrenic" of which in all my medical and personal knowledge of what was actually said, realize that the diagnosis was wrong. Doctor "X" – my first psychiatrist labeled me as having an acute psychosis – well no wonder Dr. "X" made a threatening comment which was unprofessional and I sought for other people to know about it! Here I am 30 years later trying to prove – that natural remedies are my most favored remedies and belief. In addition, a mental health diagnosis is just a diagnosis and should be met with natural ways to remedy any psychosis, delusion, etc. The environmental remedy in my case would be a good Psychologist/ therapist, understanding family/friends or psychiatrist that believes in psychotherapy without medication but interested in understanding the abuse and catastrophes I personally went through. Medication side-effects are a personal concern of mine. If I'm court ordered to take medicine, then I specifically I look for medication that doesn't cause me to be catatonic, hallucinate or be delusional. Psychotherapy would have realized that the reason I dispersed the flyers was to be heard of what happened to me. Talking about what happened is the form of therapy I choose and writing this book certainly helped!

I have since 30 years ago, spoken with therapists regarding the abuse I went through as a child, my first psychiatrist, patient in the mental health system, not being understood by family and friends, and incidence with company "Y." Physical exercise is also important to me and I work out when I can. I lift weights, do squat thrusts, and push-ups. In addition, I communicate more effectively in being understood, walk my dog for added exercise, sleep adequately, and eat healthy. I'm ideal weight and live each day trying to stay healthy. I try and maintain a spiritual balance by going to church, but also believe in GOD and things happen for a purpose generally leading to good outcomes. It is from the notion that things happen for a good reason that my spirit plays into the factor of my psyche.

Chapter Twelve

Triggers and Amends

Each time I was wrongfully petitioned then placed into an inpatient psychiatric hospital, my "delusions" which were all safe and non-threatening, began with triggers. Knowing my triggers and making amends with a difficult past certainly help in finding personal resolve and on my way to a healthy recovery. I'm currently court ordered to take psychotropic medications but have faith in someday being off a court order and will have found a solution to not being committed again into a psychiatric hospital. Part of the solution to not being committed into a psychiatric hospital is knowing what starts my delusions. My most recent wrongful inpatient psychiatric hospitalization had triggers along the way which I look back at now, and think I must amend so that I can fully recover healthily and without medication. Each trigger which culminated in another wrongful psychiatric hospitalization centered on a certain petitioner that each time misunderstood me, because of lack of communication and my most recent psychiatrist that unfortunately prescribed psychotropic medications once again as due to a court order and his neglect of not being empathetic.

The certain petitioner most often used the excuse of me not working as a result she had me committed time and time again. Now, I know her reason for petitioning me into a psychiatric hospital and can alleviate the wrongful admissions by calming this certain petitioner. I'm currently not speaking to this certain petitioner, because of her not understanding me after many times of me explaining myself and thought it would be best to just "cool off" our relationship. I plan on once again talking with the past petitioner when the time is right, in efforts to clarify things and once again build a strong relationship with understanding and her hopefully developing more empathy.

My second biggest trigger was seeing the same psychiatrist I've known in the past which spends no – more than a few minutes in talking to me during appointments. How can he know me, if he spends little time in speaking with me? – He doesn't and this particular psychiatrist triggered a delusion while in a psychiatric hospital even while having no prior recent symptoms of delusion. Knowing triggers and finding amends will certainly start a good path to personal resolve within psychiatry.

The amends I can make with this certain psychiatrist as in all my other psychiatrists that spent little time in understanding me is for me to be heard and hopefully encourage them to be more empathetic. I will let my therapist and case manager know how desperately I believe, psychiatrists have to be empathetic in efforts they may encourage them to be so as will also be therapeutic for me.

Writing this book and being heard is very important to me and it all begins with effective communication, understanding, and for empathy to be present. I'm fortunate to have discovered what my triggers are which has perpetuated themselves to lead to my delusions although safe but misunderstood. It was this misunderstanding that once again lead to many wrongful inpatient psychiatric hospitalizations. I must now expand on what I know regarding my triggers and make amends by fulfilling in doing things like writing this book so that I can be better understood, build better communication and encourage empathy in others.

Chapter Thirteen

Snowball Effect

Have you ever heard the saying "It's like a snowball going down the hill" when referring to an event? What this means is an event started, but is getting worse or better, getting bigger and bigger like a snowball rolling down a snowy hill. The negative snowball effect has been part of my life since being first involuntarily committed into a psychiatric hospital many years ago. I can now only have supervised visits with my daughter until my therapist is in agreement with my psychiatrist that I can have unsupervised visits. Both kinds of psychiatrists (hospital and psychiatric center) stated I am stable and can have supervised visits. I must now have the referral from the therapist as well saying I can have unsupervised visits with my daughter based on my inpatient involuntary psychiatric diagnosis which I know is wrong. It seems as though my experiences in mental health have led from one negative aspect to another and that I must prove myself. I had to go to court to fight for my parental Rights to see my daughter as a result of the stigma surrounding another needless psychiatric hospitalization. I represented myself, because I felt matters of the heart are best understood and expressed by the heart and I couldn't afford an attorney at the time. Unfortunately, we don't get what we want at times even in court – hoping for a more equal decision. How could they hide my true genius? I said my speech in court but still lost. It's times I wonder if I should have "bought" an attorney to represent me, but I played with my heart and I'm happy with what I said while in court but not with the result. I can live with myself knowing I mentioned in court all that I had wanted to say. I will appeal the decision for blood tests, however to determine if I'm taking the medication since I'm getting court ordered and forced injections by a nurse.

The judge handed me a life changing result and asked that I be blood tested after my court order is up to make sure that I'm still taking my medication. I thought to myself how that was infringing on my personal Rights of freedom of choice of therapy. The most natural and free from medication is truly what I requested since 30 years ago, but am still being forced to take injections.

I also thought to myself, "how could this be," after all – I only placed flyers under windshield wipers describing that I was harassed and threatened. Where's my freedom to the first amendment? I can honestly say this is the lowest point of my life, but my healthy attitude always finds the silver lining. I thought to myself I have two beautiful healthy children with having custody of my 21 year old son (since he was an adolescent), and visits with my daughter, a job I enjoy in nursing, and am physically, spiritually, and mentally healthy even though "some people" may object. I know myself more than they do and believe me, I compare my lifestyle and habits.

Time to break the chain of negative happenings in my life and can possibly kill two birds - with one stone. Writing this book may inspire people in the mental health system that are in my shoes to see the silver lining and not feel so downtrodden. In addition, I feel uplifted and exonerated in writing this book – truly therapeutic! Once again, thank you for taking your time to read this book and understand my situations better in determining the person that I truly am!

In the matter of doing the blood tests, I will inform the court that I will be receiving monthly injections as court ordered – even against my will and therefore, no blood tests are required as is my desire to be noted by the courts – finding the silver lining in a bad situation. The injections consist of alternating shots in my right and left deltoid muscles. The shot stings for a few minutes in letting the medication be pushed through the needle into my deep muscle.

I've lived most of my adult years in the psychiatric system misunderstood and was passive. It's time I let the world know that I'm intelligent and a good citizen. I played the game of keeping quiet too long. I've achieved many positive things in my life and people wonder how can I have such a good attitude with all that has happened to me? The answer is I focus on the positive attributes I have and don't let the negativity of talk by others overwhelm me.

Life truly is refreshing and joyous when I focus on the positives and with a sense of humor. My sense of humor is credited to my mother. She can be described as being "happy go lucky." Both my parents are Greek immigrants, and have taught me that perseverance and family are the most important factors of being happy and successful. I cherish each day that my parents never even thought of separating from each other and have taught that bond of togetherness to my children. I on the other hand, have been married and divorced three different times. Some of the issues that ended in divorce were that I was court ordered to take medications at some point in each of my marriages and I decided to stop taking the medication as my personal Right each time with no apparent support in tapering from my psychiatrist and developed side –effects from the abrupt stop of the medications in addition to being misunderstood and the family stress of arguing not to take medicine. I developed side effects from my medications which some made me hallucinate and be delusional. I'm now once again court ordered to take medication, because of being misunderstood and finding no time from certain family members to understand me.

The psychiatric community never once questioned Dr. "X"'s threatening remarks or how the remarks made by my manager at company "Y" affected my psyche. Both issues are of psychological aspects. I will be seeing my therapist soon, however and will talk to her about both of these aspects of which the remarks by Dr. "X" were kept a secret by me for 30 years. I did however, mention what Dr."X" had said to other professionals when it happened, but my concerns fell on deaf ears. Also, I will be speaking to more family members and friends so that I'm better understood.

Even with all the negative happenings in my life, I find happiness in myself, family, and friends. All of my family and friends are healthy and have a roof over their heads – this makes me not worry about them too much. I have since my most recent affliction being "let go" from the Family Nurse Practitioner graduate program for dispersing flyers at my clinical site, put more of my faith in GOD. I know I'm doing the best I can and help my parents and children in ways that are physically, emotionally, and spiritually healthy. Placing my faith in GOD has relinquished much stress in knowing that I'm doing all I can, and that I'm a good person that's intelligent, but misunderstood. Good things are bound to happen even more, because I have strong faith in GOD. My faith in GOD carried my son through a vehicle accident in which a salt truck skid through a stop sign and totaled his car. My son walked away from the accident with a small abrasion on his right thumb! GOD is good and we as human beings must see that there exists a spirit and GOD which gives meaning to everything and leading to positive outcomes.

I often tell myself there's a reason for everything. I enjoy helping people and with a smile am positive. Having faith in a greater purpose in helping someone else makes my own problems go away. I help my parents due to their frailness in their medical health. In fact, I work nights as a Registered Nurse so that I can take my dad to his doctor's appointments, dialysis etc. during the day. In addition, I often cook and clean for them, give my dad showers and dress him. (My dad since most recently writing the book, however refused dialysis and passed away with hospice.) My mother is more physically active than my dad and can shower and dresses herself. In addition, I prepare the pill boxes for both of my parent's medications. I only live a mile from my parents and have them on my "nanny cam" in case they need my help.

Having faith in GOD, seeing that we have a greater purpose, and knowing there are reasons for everything helps make my life whole. I live life thanking GOD for what I have and don't take anything for granted. I also, thank GOD my family and friends are healthy, live with their own autonomy and not incapacitated in a hospital bed. Being positive helps me stay focused in doing what is right and healthy for my family, friends and myself. The negative "snowball" stops here and I'm living life to the fullest as possible considering I'm court ordered to visit my therapist and case-manager once every two weeks and psychiatrist once every month and court ordered to take medication and lost parental Rights of my daughter! Being a mental health patient for 30 years (still a patient) has ruined parts of my life, because some of my family hasn't taken the time to understand me, instead they put their trust in mental health professionals which push and force medicine onto me.

I've developed a strong moral character and feel the tides are changing to a more positive outcome. Thinking positively has begun the "snowball" effect and headed in the right direction. I try and keep a positive outlook as a means to reach for what I know is right and true. Keeping positive embraces all the pleasures in life. I thank GOD that I've found the positive silver lining, and see the snowball rolling down the snowy hill getting bigger and bigger but in a positive direction through positive acts such as writing this book and being heard by more and more people. In addition, I cherish my work as a Registered Nurse, because it allows me to help others and provide a stable income for my family – another positive.

Chapter Fourteen

The Bright Spot

If I were truly psychotic I would have a much downtrodden attitude evident in my personality with all that has happened. Instead, I'm healthy mentally and physically. I realize there is a "ying" to every "yang" and now bask in what could be the positive inspiration of my life – fulfilling my life story written in this book showing that I'm me! I've lived the last 30 years of my life with the secret of my psychiatrist which made an unprofessional remark towards me and has kept me in the mental health arena after being misunderstood by family and friends in addition to side-effects from psychotropic medications. It's time for me to live my life knowing the healthy person that I am and letting other people know the real me. Many people misunderstood me as being a certain personality based on a "diagnosis" but I believe I've proved them wrong. Even my first psychiatrist 30 years ago said to me that I'm "brilliant!" I truly am picking myself up by the bootstraps, brushing the dirt off my sleeves and starting my life after being knocked down by the negatives placed on me.

It's unfortunate that people don't see the harm they can inflict by trying to convince me that I'm something that I'm not. It truly takes a person with good insight and self-reflection to see through the darkness casted over me by the wrong side of psychiatry and people trying to take advantage of my "history." I surround myself with things I appreciate doing and that makes me happy. I have also questioned myself but always lived and expressed with what my heart stated and have done no one wrong.

Being nice and helping others emotionally and physically brings satisfaction to me. I'm my parent's caretaker and have them on my "nanny cam" when I can't be with them. If it weren't for me, both my parents wouldn't be living comfortably in their own home. In fact, my dad may have even passed or be living in a nursing home while my mom would be in elderly foster care, if it weren't for my diligence in keeping them healthy with their autonomy. Could I have a mental health diagnosis and still care for my son at home, parents, father to my daughter, work as a registered nurse, and care for my dog, among all the other accomplishments I've made? It would be very difficult indeed to balance all that I have done and yet kept my sanity, if I didn't have good coping habits and was truly "chemically imbalanced" – a theory not even proven by science!

I found the positives that make me happy even after all that has happened to me. I keep my sense of humor and being nice. I thank GOD that I find the silver lining and can keep my head high. I know who I am and there is no one that can take that away from me. It does scare me at times how easily I was taken away by a petition which took me out of my own home. Being placed in a psychiatric hospital tends to lose a person's identity, but I found group discussions interesting - contributed my "two cents worth" and found it rewarding helping other patients while in the hospital. Helping others while in the psychiatric hospital even as a patient kept my identity. My identity as being a nurse professionally was shown during my efforts in talking to other patients while in group discussions. The group discussions occurred effortlessly as they did while I was a mental health worker years ago.

It took me nearly a week to open up while involuntarily committed most recently into a psychiatric hospital. For a week I stayed to myself and/or didn't contribute to group discussions because I was grieving being at the hospital. I knew that once again, I didn't need to be there and eventually opened my mind and heart in saying things that helped other people and myself emotionally and spiritually. I made many friends while in the psychiatric hospital one of which I still keep in touch with and we sometimes reminisce and joke around of our experiences while in the hospital together.

I try to keep a good and positive outlook on life. In addition, I naturally set a good role model for my kids. My family knows that I'm a diligent and caring nurse by profession that wears many hats. I also manage my parent's five rental homes and haven't thought twice about not caring for my parents. In general, I naturally keep my good person image and live by my heart guided by my mind, past and present occurrences and the will of GOD. I hold no regrets except not speaking out earlier of my difficulties experienced in psychiatry and struggles to be heard and understood. It is important for me that my family realize who I am and try to communicate with me and not place my health in the hands of the mental health system or psychiatrist.

I've worked as a registered nurse for nearly ten years and live in a middle class neighborhood. I own a car and can afford what's required to live comfortably but modestly. I enjoy staying positive, because it makes me feel young and very little do I think negative of other people. I believe in the philosophy that each person has an innate desire and yearning to live within society in being friendly and caring. Sometimes, poor circumstances and insight lead us astray, and people generally have tendencies to revert back and care for one another.

Sense of humor is also very important to me. I often look back at all the people that misunderstood me intentionally and unintentionally and can't help but laugh at the situation but at times full of anguish and frustration. I mentioned to my mental health case-manager that I was probably "one of the healthiest" men he's ever met "mentally and physically!" My case-manager just looked at me with a blank look on his face and didn't say anything until our next topic of discussion. I've learned to laugh at many of my life instances, because if I didn't laugh then I would cry.

At least, the first psychiatrist – Dr. "X" and myself are in agreement about one thing – that I'm "brilliant!" It's interesting how I remember each of my encounters that happened, which started nearly 30 years ago with a psychiatrist that took so much away from me, and close family.

If you recall as I mentioned in previous chapters, Dr. "X" labeled me as having an "acute psychosis" in relation to me trying to break out of a psychiatric unit from his unprofessional and threatening remark. I threw the chair at the window when I was 19 years old to make a point of how unprofessional the psychiatrist was not that I truly believed he was going to harm me. The label of "paranoid schizophrenia" stuck from other doctors thinking I hallucinated what Dr. "X" had said!

The bright spot in all my years of being misunderstood by psychiatry and had family that carelessly didn't care to find out the real me, but instead depended on psychiatry and the mental health system is that I haven't lost insight of the real me! I unfortunately am keeping on taking my medication, because the courts have mandated that I do and I basically can't have unsupervised visits with my daughter unless the order changes in relation to a psychiatric diagnosis. I would much rather have talk therapy in place of taking medication. I appreciate the readers in taking the time to "listen" to what I have to say. Writing this book has been therapeutic for me and I hope for you as well.

I found that forcing someone as myself to take medication is a form of control by the other group of people and is oppression. They believe by forcing me to take medication that I won't be distributing flyers. This sort of control they have over me by forcing me to take medications also involves seeing a therapist to talk about my concerns and psychiatrist to help manage my medication. Hence, the group involvement once again centered on taking medication. The bright spot again, is that I still feel healthy and am happy being "me." I've noticed some medication side-effects such as extensive cotton mouth especially while sleeping, and occasional involuntary muscle movements. My Right of the first amendment was also breached – the freedom of speech. Why is my Right to disperse flyers taken away from me? Is it "mentally ill" to let the public know what happened to me 30 years ago yet have no resolve? The bright spot here is that I know myself to be happy and am surrounding myself with individuals that have also been injured by psychiatry as a form of group therapy. In addition, family and friends are better understanding me – another bright spot, perhaps the brightest.

I'm finding outlets such as Facebook, blogs and reading books with individuals that have been harmed by psychiatry as a form of release and form of expressing myself. I realize my life story is confusing and even difficult to understand, but it must be told so that other people may realize they are not alone in their struggles with psychiatry, losing Rights and forced into treatment, and to be understood. Hopefully, people will have found some inspiration after reading this book in being who they want to be and not letting negative talk or misunderstanding get in their way of reaching their full potential and happiness. Happiness is subjective to each of us and I urge the reader to pick your battles and fight the good fight when you're ready. For me, initiating the fight to be understood started with the power mostly by trying to be heard as now through describing the real me and not what psychiatry wants me, friends, or family to believe.

Chapter Fifteen

Freedom of Speech

My flyers written regarding dispute with company "Y" had no violence in them, they merely stated how I was harassed, and threatened while working there then "let go." I understand it's been nearly 21 years ago, but there was no resolve and I was left with reaching out so that I could be heard. As I mentioned earlier, the only therapy I will agree to and not forced to do is talk therapy, however appropriate socialization with family and friends is the most important. I would like to explore the threatening remark by Dr. "X" which kept me in the realm of psychiatry for 30 years and what happened at company "Y." My flyers and picket signs were a method of me coping with what had happened in the past. Not many people realize how my life was scarred by what the doctor said and what happened to me while working for company "Y."

The flyers and picket signs in a sense were my method to "talk" about what happened and find someone to share what had occurred. I have a therapist which, I see but will mention to her my frustrations with both situations regarding Doctor "X" and company "Y." I was merely too carried away with how my Rights were abridged from me, everyday life experiences, and secrets of what happened, to talk to my therapist about what truly bothered me. Writing this book has helped in many ways to release pinned up frustrations and described the secrets in my life which have caused misunderstanding and havoc and resulted in unnecessary inpatient psychiatric hospitalizations, because people didn't make efforts in trying to understand me. Instead, petitions once again kept creeping up and unnecessarily had me committed into psychiatric hospitals.

In a sense, writing this book is like talk therapy. I feel a good release of emotions in writing my thoughts in book form. The nurse side of me also appreciates this book in thinking that I may be helping someone else in the same circumstance as I'm having or have society be more empathetic toward people involved in the mental health arena. The events that surround hospital admissions, petitions, involuntary inpatient psychiatric hospitalizations, being misunderstood, and forced treatments have been a part of my life for the last 30 years. It feels good in knowing that I'm having therapy in writing this book and being a nurse in helping other people by describing events which they may also learn from and hopefully not repeat.

Chapter Sixteen

Family and Companionship

The importance of good social interactions helps the soul to find happiness and reassurance. Being understood by family is probably one of the most important aspects in my life right now. Time and time again a certain family member carelessly and absentmindedly placed my mental health in the hands of a psychiatrist and the mental health system without taking the time to understand me. I'm convinced that if family took the time to understand me, then I wouldn't have spent one minute in a psychiatric hospital. Fortunately, for me I made a friend in a psychiatric hospital whom I still share time with.

Making a friend in the psychiatric hospital gave me more purpose in being there. Purpose driven activities help me to relax and find pleasure in life. My children are important to me as is standing up for my Rights. It is difficult for anyone to fathom the complex circumstances I've witnessed, but one thing I've never lost sight of was a sense of myself and the importance of sharing my thoughts, aspirations and feelings with someone close.

I've learned to be with people that make me happy, understand me as a person - and not someone that has merely a diagnosis in the psychiatric realm. It's difficult at times knowing what I've gone through and carrying the label as being a "paranoid schizophrenic," but I don't let that bother me much at all, because I know my self-proclamation of being healthy – my Psychologist said I'm "normal" and that my symptoms are a result of psychiatric abuse. Even my psychiatrists say I'm stable and "brilliant." True companionship is finding peace within yourself and those around you.

Sometimes a person must realize that they have gone over their head and need to step back and reflect or just be separated from the life stress. I chose to work in an acute care hospital to challenge myself and find my strength knowing what my weaknesses may already be. I found myself excelling on being a floor nurse then charge nurse, preceptor and mentor.

Challenge is good in that it allows for growth. Social relationships also make me find the special hat, but depending on who you're with you can either look like a fool or just plain enjoy yourself and be you. I've learned we can't change people's attitudes towards us, but we may be able at times to persuade their thoughts about who we are. Being a nurse has helped me play the role of care provider, comedian, teacher, technician, and many other personalities in wearing different hats.

I have found that immature people can make you look like an idiot by gaslighting and even lying about your character. Unfortunately, not everyone has a broad knowledge base and empathy when speaking to other people. I've always been a kind person and that at times doesn't work in my favor. I've learned there are people in this world which take advantage of kind people to see how far they can take the person's limit. This sort of "pushing" the other person's "buttons" can either be contended with apprehension, fear, or passivity.

I have been passive most of my life but determined enough is enough and have constructively let people know when they have pushed my buttons one too many times. It is important to notify the other person's intrusion because, if not they will keep being aggressive and try to control your life. Unfortunately, having the experience of being committed multiple times into a psychiatric hospital involuntarily carries a stigma of being thought of as thinking unclearly and unstable. Many people in my life have taken advantage of the stigma of prior hospitalizations and carelessly set my true character aside. I unfortunately, can't change the attitudes of some people towards me, but have determined that if they act negatively towards me it's because of their own ignorance. My lesson in life is to be around people that understand you and make you happy.

I was taught to treat people how they treat you, however I've found it within myself to set a good example rather than get even. I base a lot of my actions on my morals that way I have no regrets. I let my heart and mind guide my actions and try to do what's right. It's too easy to get back at someone, but my moral character tries to reach above the belittling of each other. I have less personal stress and guilt if I treat people genuinely.

Who is to say or intervene in my personal affairs? The person I met while in the psychiatric hospital was stigmatized with people's thoughts related to a person being "mentally ill." I didn't appreciate how short sighted people in public were with my friend I had met in the psychiatric hospital. Unfortunately, stigma is real and people that do stigmatize are the last to admit of their moral crime criticizing other people. I try not to dwell on what other people think, however it is not assuring knowing that certain people act on their short sighted beliefs and close off learning about other people. When the short sightedness begins to affect how they interact with the person they have negative thoughts about is when it's a concern of my personal feelings and thoughts.

Chapter Seventeen

Passivity

Being passive has its benefits of not getting too involved in stressful situations, but enough is enough! I will truly be a slave to whoever is in my path, if I continue being passive. I've determined it's time to obtain what my children and I deserve – righteousness! I've been mister nice guy for all my life and now I want something more. I've determined a keen way to let the world know of how much I'd like to change the psychiatric system and issues I have with certain people, the freer I will be. It seems as though being nice allowed too many people to take advantage of my passive ways.

A good first step for me in becoming free with less stress is to express my thoughts to people that I think will be empathetic. After all, you can talk to someone, but if you don't believe they will be empathetic, then you're wasting your time. It's difficult to choose the right person to talk to, because you believe they will change but chances are some people probably won't. I can't stress enough how important it is to pick the person you believe will share your beliefs. There comes a time when you would like to change someone's mind but take it with a grain of salt, because you can only try to change the opinion of some people some time. Other people just don't have the empathy and fortitude to grasp what is said so don't be surprised if they may never get your point. You know what they say "You can take a horse to water but you can't make him drink." The people I'm trying to make my points across to are once again, the same ones that neglected my feelings and thoughts for many years.

Challenging yourself, however can also make you free once you overcome the obstacle. There is a delicate balance between knowing when to surround yourself with empathetic people and when to surround yourself with people that may challenge your beliefs. I've learned a little challenge every once in a while stimulates change. Change may be good sometimes. Don't underestimate the power of a good challenge, but know when you're over your head and start to make amends with your thoughts. Don't put too many challenges close together without some kind of self-reflection to keep insight of who you are.

Passivity has the other benefit of staying out of trouble, so if you're just getting started on voicing your opinion then take it slow. The most pleasurable aspect of life is being free and living life how you want. Remember to smell the roses and always put being nice at the top of your list. How you treat people is how you would like to be treated. We all lose our cool sometimes, but remember that occurrence should be a rare entity. People can understand a genuine individual and respect their nature. One of the best ways to get back at your enemies is to succeed. Plan on winning and remember to plan ahead on staying cool. Even through all that I have gone through – the many involuntary wrongful commitments into psychiatric hospitals, being misunderstood, and forced treatments, I still kept my cool and am nice. Refreshing and true was the comment by the custody case judge when he finished the court hearing by saying "John you're a kind man." He also said "Good luck with your mental health struggles." – He knew that I had a lot to say and fighting the system that took so much away from me and close family which left me without psychological reference was soon to be my next aim in life. I felt as though I needed to have some retribution and exoneration from an oppressive mental health system. I always stayed who I am – a nice guy. I've been asked "Why are you so nice?" I replied "Because that's me and it makes me happy."

Perhaps what keeps me happy is that when I look back, I try and learn from my mistakes and mistakes around me, but I don't let them get me down. Coping strategies help, but another big influence is keeping physically active, spiritually happy, and eating healthy. I find happiness in everything I do but, if I'm not physically or emotionally fit then it's difficult to stay healthy. I'm fortunate to have a dog I can walk with, if I have the urge to enjoy a brisk walk through the neighborhood. My advice with regards to being active is find an exercise you enjoy and perform it at least three days during the week for thirty minutes each day. Sometimes you may alter your routine, but still find the happiness in doing whatever you're doing. You may also find an intense exercise such as a burpee which is a modified squat thrust and perform it for two minutes which gives you the same benefits as a 40 minute moderate work out.

It's easy to get caught up in the hustle and bustle of the day but find time for yourself and live life to be happy. Keep in tune with who you are and don't let anyone else command your feelings. Stay away from people that don't empathize. Remember, it's okay to break away from the passive shell we all sometimes find refuge in keeping ourselves emotionally safe.

It's easier said than done when determining when to be passive as opposed to needing a good challenge. Let change be the trigger to determine which you'd like in your life – being passive or looking for a challenge. You will never know your full potential, if you don't challenge yourself. Sometimes your enemy could be your best friend. Open your eyes to new possibilities and have a good sense of who you are and what you're capable of achieving. It's also a good practice to learn how to pick your battles and try not to get too involved with the present when there's a dispute you know at the time - you may not succeed. You can always come back to an argument. Also remember, it's better to make friends than enemies. Being passive has the benefit to help control your emotions, but sometimes you have to express what you truly believe.

Chapter Eighteen

Medicated for Society's Delusions and Anxieties

My life story is so twisted that I must be medicated to pacify society because it becomes delusional into thinking that I must be medicated to function properly. It seems as though I can continue stating my life story using means of communication such as writing books and stating what is wrong and not be committed into a psychiatric hospital if I take my medication as a way to pacify the community. It's like a green light allowing me to continue stating my resolve and not be involuntarily committed. I could always think clearly except when having side effects to certain psychotropic medications. I strongly believe as what I personally went through is that psychiatry is made to pacify society, psychiatrists and even careless family members that don't take the time to realize and understand the "patient." Medication for me was a way to pacify the petitioner and the mental health system. The mental health system I found is very oppressive with the end result forcing people to take medicine.

It's kind of ironic in thinking that I'm free because I can express myself but only when court ordered to take medications because the people that committed me believe I'm being taken care of by psychiatry if I take the medicine. I'm so disgusted with what psychiatry has done to me and close family which left me with writing my concerns while mandating me by the court to be drugged through psychotropic medications.

Psychiatry hasn't done anything right for me and has caused me grief. It seems as though the psychiatric patient is treated even less than a criminal in thinking they can't determine what's right for themselves while even many times losing their Rights and being involuntarily committed into a psychiatric hospital. How can I let the psychiatric professionals know that I'm healthy if they take away my tools to prove that I'm sane? For instance, I showed my psychiatrist awards that I received as an undergraduate and graduate student including scholarships, honor certificates and even nurse of the year awards. He stated mental health is indifferent to intelligence. Does he not understand that to be a nurse you must have all your faculties? Also, to be an honor student you need to be consistently good at thinking clearly! Psychiatry has proven itself to me that it's oppressive.

I believe that I'm medicated through court order to pacify society and of which was never needed. Psychiatrists and therapists have too much say in what is "best for the patient." The psychiatrists and therapists I've personally been involved in, lacked empathy of my true feelings and thoughts. They believed what they wanted to believe so that I fit their profile of what a "mentally ill" patient is like.

The medication I'm taking is given to me I believe to pacify society into thinking everything is "okay" now thanks to the psychiatrist which is disgusting and revolting. My treatment in mental health has left me with grief, despair, and animosity towards mental health professionals and even family members that haven't taken the time to talk with me in understanding my thoughts and feelings. I thank GOD that I can provide my services of being a kind and caring man through being a nurse and personal life of caring for my family. The evil doings of psychiatry can't take away the fact that I perform good deeds at work and in my personal life. Unfortunately, and regrettably psychiatry is trying to get the credit of my good deeds by making the public believe that I'm "being treated" and am being a good citizen, because I'm taking (court ordered) psychotropic medicine. I've always been a good citizen and even a "do - gooder" throughout my life with or without psychotropic medications.

Chapter Nineteen

Being a Registered Nurse is Being Me

We all have our graces in keeping ourselves sane and mine is being a nurse. I thank GOD that I have my job, because it allows me to be me! Being a nurse requires empathy, patience, knowledge, desire to do no harm, encouraging others, and self to be healthy. What more in a career could I want? People look at me and can't believe I've been committed into a psychiatric hospital multiple times "You look and act so normal" they say, well guess what I AM normal but have been a part of the mental health system which lacks empathic doctors and had deleterious side effects to medicine as well as not being understood by family and friends due to nearly non-existent communication! I never let anyone else tell me what I'm not. After all I know myself better than anyone. No one should have the power to judge anyone else yet most of my adult life was spent being judged by others. The multiple involuntary psychiatric commitments caused stigma in my life towards me, because people automatically assumed that I'm short sided, hallucinatory, and delusional. Actions speak louder than words and it seems as though people go out of their way to "error on being safe" when interacting with someone with a mental health condition. My character soon makes people relax, because I think they realize that I'm not the monster they envisioned me as being before talking to me. Mental health stigma is prevalent in our society. Even some of my therapists were influenced with people's misperceptions of a "mentally ill" person as I've noticed myself being misunderstood. Unless you stand up for yourself, people will automatically assume you as their own preconceived notion and many times has negative connotations. I'd like for a particular family member to get to know me, because she spent no time in trying to understand my "delusions" which were caused by psychotropic medications, and/or an unresolved distraught past, but instead she had me taken away and "cared for" by the hands of mental health "professionals."

I figure the best time is now to let people know that I'm still successful after all that I've been through – the wrongful psychiatric admissions and petitions which took me away from my friends and family. Amen! For all that I have. I feel blessed and will continue on being me! I chose the right profession and I dare say that if I didn't have my registered nurse license, I'd still be me! I believe people see me as being authentic and genuine after talking with me. If a person believes me to have good character and qualities, then they've found me. I'm truly empathetic when talking to people and that is a quality I recognize in other people as well.

It helps to stay positive, and that I believe is also a good quality of being me and a nurse. Staying positive is close to my other quality of being optimistic. Always finding reason to "make it through" has made me successful. I have chosen to write this book to help exonerate people that have been misunderstood by so many in the psychiatric field. It makes me proud to be a nurse, but even more proud knowing that I'm no longer passive in trying to make myself believe in something that I'm not. Finding my new role and purpose in life is exciting and a "cake walk," because I'm me and I know who I am. I'm not a label and I have feelings and emotions like everyone else. I've been in the medical/psychiatric field as a "patient" and professional for many years and know human emotions well enough to self-proclaim and justify my thoughts about who I am. I think standing up for what a nurse is, is standing up for myself!

Writing is proof that talk therapy through communication helps me realize who I am and of my potential. Being a nurse shines through the darkness and leads me to finding the bright side. Authoring this book was a good remedy to a wounded soul much like washing with soap and water is to an open wound.

Chapter Twenty

Why the Fuss?

People often ask me, why are you making such a big deal out of a label? My answer is that I wouldn't care so much, if it meant that my Rights to choose how I wanted to live my life weren't jeopardized. I've lost my Right to the type of treatment I should have and am fighting for parental rights of my daughter all due to a psychiatric diagnosis and stigma of being a mental health patient. The turmoil I'm in is based on being caught up in the stigma of mental health. I didn't do anyone wrong but voiced my concerns. I was never a threat to myself or others but "fell through the cracks" and wrongfully placed into a psychiatric hospital many times. Now, I'm once again court ordered into treatment. The court order stated that I must be on medication and under the guidance of a psychiatrist for another six months. I live my life as close to being natural as possible and believe in holistic methods. Can you empathize with me knowing that I'd like to heal myself? Each time I acted in ways to express myself, I was met with a petition pick-up order then evaluated by a psychiatrist to be committed into a psychiatric hospital due to "falling through the cracks" again. I had no say in how I'd be treated and even acted upon - like I was a criminal. Clearing my name and breaking away from a system that has forced its ways upon me and caused harm seems the logical thing to do. I'm 49 years old and have struggled with the mental health system since I was 19 years old. I've been passive and submissive for all those years and it's done nothing, but kept me in the mental health arena and even forced me into treatment along with developing personal stress, anguish, and duress. I wish to be let go and keep me free from coming back. I've just now gotten the courage to explain the secrets that I've kept for so many years and decided to break free from a system that has created misunderstandings, involuntary admissions to psychiatric hospitals, forced outpatient therapies, and time away from my family, and friends.

Another bigger reason for the fuss is trying to bring my family back together. A certain family member chose to allow the mental health "professionals" in attempting to heal me as opposed to getting to know why I may have been "delusional" or had a "psychosis." Even, to this day I resent ever my involvement as a patient in mental health and how I'd like to sit down with family away from mental health professional influences. Getting to know me away from medicine will surely know me best. I often, wish I would have had many long conversations with family long ago so that they knew me and not be forced into "treatment."

The human mind is strong and resilient. I've witnessed my life misunderstood and have been passive. Like a doormat I let psychiatric professionals rule my life and have witnessed wrongful petitions and hospitalizations. In the face of all the adversarial instances, I've come on top in making my point. I've presented myself well during my undergraduate and graduate level classes and completed my assignments in the top 5% of my class. It's going to take a book such as this to help clarify who I really am as opposed to a person that has been involuntarily committed into multiple psychiatric hospitals and with all its negative connotations. A book such as this explaining that what I need most is to sit with family and friends and talk with them so that they get to know me and I get to know them more.

If I don't try and clarify who I am, then these needless hospitalizations which have taken so much away from me and my family will continue as will misunderstanding my personality. Clarifying who I am will also bring back my personal identity, and not who other people are trying to make me believe I am. I try to keep a sense of humor so that I may relieve stress. It's easy for me to laugh at myself, but people judge each other every day and I can't help but think that I had the "short end of the stick" one too many times.

The stigma of mental health unfortunately carries itself especially with people involuntarily committed in psychiatric hospitals such as myself. I don't let the stigma personally bother me, because I know what may be thought of me is not true. I live with a clear conscience in saying what is true. I've stated my life story without being false and gave credit where it's due.

Clarifying who I am will help bring resolve to my past which is something no one or any involvement in any system has done for me so far. Being middle aged has its benefits of being heard more intently and empathetically especially by those younger than I am. One of the most important things in my life now is to have a sense of resolve from my past so that I can move forward. I've always known that I was "normal" but had difficulties in explaining myself, because it seemed as if my concerns always fell on deaf ears and had things manifest with "delusions" and even hallucinations as a result of no resolve, being misunderstood and side-effects to medicine.

Making resolve with my past is similar to knowing where I'm going now that the past is behind me. I've learned in life that sometimes I can't move forward without fixing the present or healing from the past. Also, I'd like my children and any future grandchildren to know the real me, especially if there are any mental health – medical questions they may have. I've mentioned many things through writing in this book that will help friends and relatives make their own conclusions of as to my character, mental state, and present field of psychiatric help. I hope they see me as the authentic and genuine person that I truly am.

It feels good to finally make my own identity and not struggle with a label I know is confusing to say the least. I've identified myself for the first time in 30 years by describing secrets that I've kept bottled inside me since a very young man entering adulthood. I'm recognizing my scars and finding ways to cope with and resolve the past. Hopefully, I can say that I've succeeded in standing my ground to the stigma of mental health, people sabotaging my character, and in clarifying who I am when I look back from the next 30 years of my life.

Another accomplishment I wish to make is making myself heard in the psychiatric field so that psychiatry recognizes changes need to be made. I know from personal contacts in organizations that other people have similar stories as mine. People that were passive are starting to speak up against a system that is oppressive and harmed them. The type of harm in psychiatry may be physical as through forced treatments or psychological through coercion and oppression. People that are in positions within the medical field and have been wronged are obligated to voice their concerns so that the more vulnerable people that can't speak for themselves will be heard. Public awareness of a faulty system is the first step in resolving issues especially involving human Rights, treatment options, personal, and social affairs.

It's time for psychiatry to realize people are talking and wish to see changes which will benefit the patient and not error on the side of being safe while jeopardizing patient human Rights. It saddens me to think my amendment of freedom of speech was taken away and then tried to pacify me through harmful medications and non-empathetic psychiatrists. I'd rather live free under my own guise and not forced treatment against my beliefs. I hope mental health professionals will realize that the patient knows best of their own condition and please listen to what the patients are saying about what may be wrong in the mental health system or treatment they are having or experiencing and do something positive to change the system.

People that wonder why I make all the fuss have probably never had their Rights mistakenly taken away or been misunderstood to the extent it causes mental anguish, stress, and duress. It's difficult to see the world as I do, and I'm glad not many people see the non-empathetic, controversial therapies, and time away from family and friends while confined involuntarily in a psychiatric hospital or forced outpatient treatment. People exist however, that wish to see changes and more people are evident in doing so. I believe psychiatry will soon see changes in how diagnoses are made and hopefully rule against taking away human Rights. Any person would fight for their freedom and I'm no different. The next time I'm asked "why the fuss? I'll answer - wars were fought over loss of freedom. I've always believed in resolving issues with civility and never once condoned violence.

Breaking the string of involuntary commitments into psychiatric hospitals is another goal in writing this book and identifying the real me. If I don't speak up, it sets me up for another unnecessary psychiatric hospitalization. Standing up for myself will help send a clear message that I shouldn't be hospitalized. Even if I were misunderstood and hospitalized again I'd write another chapter in my book, because the right and just ways prevail. I act upon what I do the right way so that I play with a clear conscience and give credit where it's due. I know what I deserve, and living a life how I would like with outside intervention telling me what I can and can't do is not what I planned. Not taking medication is not negotiable at this point, because of the wrongful court order and may not be for a long time. Another judge in custodial parent court ordered that I take medicine, if I'd like to have unsupervised visitations with my daughter. At least writing this book describes who I am, and makes my points clear in helping psychiatry and people harmed by it. The most recent harm aside from my psychological psyche and possible medication side-effects, is that of infringement on my Rights to live how I'd like to live without medications and outpatient psychiatric involvement.

Living my life how I intend to live is my goal. I will make sacrifices, however such as taking the court ordered medication to see my daughter. If I must take medication then I will continue taking that which I'm on, because of it currently not having any noticeable side –effects, except for occasional lower jaw and right hand tremors, but hesitate to wonder the long term effects of the medication. I enjoy being a father, relative, son, friend, and nurse but being set up for future failure by not standing up for myself will no longer be personally tolerated.

I will stand up for myself and be heard. I know I've turned some heads with my statements and they are all true, but changes would be much appreciated and necessary. My only regret is not standing up for myself sooner. As I mentioned before, there is a reason for everything and the reason is now. Since I must currently take the medication and continue with outpatient treatment as court ordered, I will find within myself to keep identifying who I truly am. It is very easy for someone to succumb into thinking they are someone whom they are not while part of the mental health system, because our concerns too often fall on deaf ears and many professionals are not empathetic. As more and more people have been hurt by psychiatry and speaking out, the mental health system will hopefully listen to our concerns and make positive changes.

The next step in making changes is finding a venue where patients and psychiatric staff can meet and exchange thoughts. More credence and credit must also be given to the patient and not merely be submissive or passive anymore. Psychiatry needs to be more aware of the concerns people are having. There are many concerns as already stated which have caused stress on patients wrongfully committed into psychiatric hospitals.

Chapter Twenty-One

Jack in a Box

Stigma leads into being misunderstood. I know myself as being healthy but responding to stressful situations in a way that may make me appear to have a mental health condition or a result to coming off psychotropic medicine too quickly or side-effects to medicine or misunderstood by family. Stigma and being misunderstood stand together. The stigma of being involuntarily committed into a psychiatric hospital many times conjures up thoughts that are negative and submissive brought on by a system that is oppressive and coercive. I'm often amused in talking to people that know I've been hospitalized and listen to things that they believe may be wrong with me. It's funny to note that what they thought of - such as at times that I'm being forgetful or making "poor decisions" concerning a "significant other" are forms of being "mentally ill." I can't help but laugh at how normal I am when people describe me as being "mentally ill." We all are forgetful at times and sometimes let our heart guide us with decisions of whom we choose to be with as our significant other. People live their life many times under certain circumstances which make our life difficult at times. Difficult times sometimes makes people forgetful and in making poor decisions due to stress, anguish, and duress. It's interesting to note that I'm still with my close "significant other," of which I met in the psychiatric hospital. I sometimes, however feel like a Jack in a box as if I were everyone's side-kick, because of being labeled as "mentally ill." It seems as though the definition of being "mentally ill" gets redefined for the purpose of someone having a sort of control over a "patient" individual or are just plain careless with intent to hurt someone's character or feelings. I believe it goes back to human nature – the negative thoughts people have of each other are to mask our own insecurities.

I believe it's human nature to automatically take something as how it is presented in front of you without question. For instance, very few people scrutinize the information they have or know of about someone else and believe in hearsay. I question everything about people, especially what is said to me about them and often times give them benefit of the doubt in proving their good qualities. A goal in writing this book is for people to question what they know and think of other possibilities in helping their cause. There are many people that also think with a one track mind, and can't empathize or see the other person's point of view. I've found these kind of people to be judgmental and often times high strung. It is unfortunate that even certain members of my own family haven't taken the time to get to know me and time and time again it was dependent on an outside source – psychiatrists to try and make sense of my condition. Each time I met with a psychiatrist, it was the worst thing that could happen to me because they didn't talk to explore more about me they just went by what the petitioner said and prescribed medicine! The medicine and lack of psychiatrist's insight in who I am caused me an enormous amount of anguish, stress, and duress.

Exploring other people's feelings and thoughts creates empathy and a genuine wholeness. I believe I would make a good therapist – if that were my intentions, because I know the value of psychotherapy and can empathize. I thank GOD for my sense of humor in dealing with people that can't see my point of view. My mind is flexible and can handle someone that grossly misinterprets me except until it's reached this point where I must express myself due to all of the negativity I've witnessed due to psychiatry and not being heard by my family. Perhaps I've learned to cope with people that don't see my point of view, because I hope they will eventually learn to view my opinions and comments. People that know me realize that I'm very patient, quiet, and certainly not forgetful. I realize this is a form of being passive, submissive, but I'm working on letting my point of view be known.

Writing this book and coalescing my research paper are good starts to making people understand the "difficulties" of our current mental health system and the struggles a person may have on the wrong side of psychiatry.

I will admit it's difficult creating a new identity that's been passive and submissive - most years of my adult life. I've determined that if I don't state my point of view then people will automatically assume the most negative qualities as conjured from being involuntarily (wrongfully) committed into psychiatric hospitals. I have found that people which view me as being passive and submissive have the greater tendency of treating me like a doormat and walk all over my emotions. I can tell a person that can truly empathize and sees the real me. I believe the next step I should take is being polite when voicing my opinion in talking to other people. This should be easy, because I'm polite and genuine by nature. In fact, I think what many people will say about me is that I'm a good listener and help people with their own problems. Part of being a nurse is taking in information that is known then helping others after carefully making an assessment of what may be wrong.

I can't be the Jack in the box my entire life. Expressing my feelings more as in writing and talking to people is a sort of life changer re-birth. Hopefully, people will recognize the hardships I've had through all the stigma and misunderstandings, then begin to ask me questions. Replying to questions and carrying on a conversation will reveal that I'm more like the other person than they previously believed and not a preconceived "mental health patient." I'm finally waking up to the fact of how misunderstood I've been by most people of my adult life. I figure that I have the rest of my life to show that I'm not the preconceived person people believe I am – at least not from the stigma of having been committed unnecessarily involuntarily into psychiatric hospitals, because I was misunderstood.

I think the key to opening up - for me, is talking to people and encouraging them to ask questions. The more a person knows me, the more they will realize similarities between us. I'm human and seek in other people what they seek in me. I think people would like someone that is honest and not afraid to constructively tell them what is wrong. I hope after reading this book, that the medical psychiatric profession will also open their eyes and make changes to psychiatry and be more empathetic. Being passive has its benefits, but sometimes breaking out from my shell creates positive circumstances. I look forward to how people will perceive me. I no longer plan on being passive or submissive, but voice my concerns through writing books and possibly even public speaking.

It's time to explore what it's like to project a positive self-image knowing that other people may have prejudged me from being in a psychiatric hospital. I enjoy being me and will continue doing what I do to improve the mental health system and voice my personal concerns of being misunderstood. I've also come to the realization that people may be wondering what's wrong with me and I can't help but say - nothing, but gone through extreme stress, anguish and duress then having my mind play tricks on me – a normal response to emotional trauma and being misunderstood. I believe my childhood friends that know me best would like to see me break out from my shell as well. I think they would like the struggle they perceive me going through to be over and I win trying to make my points of psychiatry being more empathetic and open their mind to new possibilities. I also believe my friends would like to see me be exonerated from the mental health system that took so much away from me, close family, and friends. I have much to offer in a personality that truly cares, has good understanding, and a sense of humor. A person's personality can tell a lot about a person, but we must not forget that circumstances often times creates an environment that may not necessarily allow the person to express their true thoughts and feelings. This book was an important tool and in letting the public know the real me and hopefully will inspire changes within an ailing mental health system.

Chapter Twenty-Two

Coercion

Psychiatry is oppressive with the psychiatrist's diagnosis apparently being the final say in how a patient gets treated and not the patient's, as was with my personal experience, I had little if any say in how I wanted to be treated assuming I wanted to be treated. I felt as though from day one in seeing a psychiatrist that I was coerced into the medication regimen of psychiatry. Psychiatrists unfortunately have the power to write letters with their diagnosis and beliefs of how "safe" an individual is or can be in society. They unfortunately mention their diagnosis erroring on "being safe" even though the patient's Rights or personal temperament of how they truly are is being jeopardized. The wrongful interpretation of how a patient truly is by the psychiatrist or other mental health professional, is a form of mental abuse.

The psychiatrist or any mental health professional can't be with a patient all the time or truly determine what they are thinking. It is this knowing, that psychiatrists and mental health care professionals can't be with the patients all the time or know what they are truly saying that makes psychiatry a subjective field, because there are no lab or blood tests to determine brain chemistry, it makes psychiatry a truly subjective field of medicine and not even a true science.

It is unfortunate that I feel as though I must be submissive and compliant with treatment even though I'm strongly against the medications. I must abide by the psychiatrist's plan of care of medication because psychiatry today is all about the doctor prescribing medications and psychiatric oppression.

There exists a tremendous amount of duress against patients that are under the "care' of a psychiatrist. We must follow the straight path of "treatment" or determined to be "non-compliant." The most coercive propaganda portrayed by my psychiatrist is that I was told that

I must take my medications in order for my psychiatrist and therapist to write a letter stating that they will allow me to have unsupervised visits with my daughter!

The stigma of being determined "mentally ill" in child custody court regarding parenting time was real. There was a time recently when I had to go to court and fought for more parenting time but the stigma of being determined "mentally ill" made the judge decide that I must take my medication in order for me to have unsupervised visits with my daughter. The stigma of mental health, social ignorance, cruelty, a mental health system that errors on being safe but jeopardizing human Rights, a failed psychiatric system and people being short sighted have ruined parts of my adult life!

I have found that psychiatry is run helter-skelter with little to no empathy for the patient. Even though psychiatry has no scientific basis its pretended to be of the same caliber as medical science of which of course, is not. I have also found that psychiatry is like a police state pretending to do society a favor or drugging the patient so that they may not "act out." Psychiatry animalizes its patients into doing what the psychiatrist has conjured. Often times, as was my personal experience, psychiatrists don't even ask what the patient is believing. Not one time in my 30 years of involuntarily being a mental health patient, did a psychiatrist ask me what I was thinking! The psychiatrist only played on what he/she thought would be the "safest" thing to do not even knowing my good moral character and basing their judgements off what the petitioner stated even gaslighting ways! My Rights were taken away many times in the name of psychiatry and what is even as troubling is the fact that I was treated like an animal and coerced into taking medications against my will and unnecessarily meeting with a therapist every two weeks for two years in a row – on several occasions but with time periods varying. Equally troubling is that I was forced to pay for the medication, psychiatrist, and therapist using my own medical insurance of which thankfully was Medicaid but soon to be stopped due to my income.

It is truly sad that the psychiatrists in all my years' experience as an involuntary mental health patient wrongfully hospitalized, never once explored my thoughts. One of the main reasons why I became recommitted into psychiatric hospitals was to be heard of the terrible injustices in my life including being mistreated by mental health professionals especially psychiatrists. Talking to psychiatrists has been very difficult because they focus on one thing and that's medications. I have a personal belief of not having to take medicine and being forced to take medicine is against my belief but the psychiatrist's and therapist's coercion in making me take medications in order for me to see my daughter, is a fear of the repercussions that may occur by mental health professionals and custody court, if I don't take my medications. Times are changing and I'm making my points known and hope that someday the truth will set me free and people will better understand me and the doctor will notice that all I ever needed was to talk with someone that was empathetic and be understood away from the prescriptive medical model.

Chapter Twenty-Three

Making Resolve and Amends

I've described many personal afflictions I've suffered from being misunderstood and a victim of psychiatry. This chapter will focus on making amends to the turmoil I've suffered along with close family and friends. There are suggestions I've thought of in making amends, and they all will be resolved through more quality social interactions. These social interactions will hopefully encourage the people in question of petitioning me to realize my positive qualities and directive of never wanting to be a mental health patient especially not to be seen again by a psychiatrist!

Close family and friends are important to me, therefore I will attempt in making amends with the people that have misunderstood me for the majority of the last 30 years! Also, I believe in forgiving to better live a holistic life without carrying the toxic abuse I've suffered in the last 30 years of my life being a mental health patient by certain people in my past. I plan on forgiving the people that petitioned me several times in the past into psychiatric hospitals, but not forgetting the hardships they caused. I will, however open up to talking and socializing more with the people that have misunderstood me for so many years. I believe them understanding me, and talking will once again create a more copacetic environment in preventing misunderstanding which wrongfully led to inpatient psychiatric hospitalizations.

I've learned that company "Y" and doctor "X" will probably not ever seek to make resolve with me as I've tried many times for them to even speak with me as I personally attempted to visit them. In addition, I've learned to fill the void of no real resolve with company "Y" or doctor "X" with the knowing that more people are listening to my story and that I don't have to place flyers under windshield wipers or picket company entrances anymore.

I would like to once again thank you for reading this book, because it truly makes me content knowing my life story is being heard in efforts to make better amends. Once again, thank you. I feel as though my points are being made and now am ready to move onto the next stage of my life and seek/make resolve with the people that have done me and my close family/friends wrong for so many years. Once again, thank you.

Chapter Twenty-Four

Betrayed by Psychiatry

I have personally witnessed for 30 years that psychiatrists don't take the time to listen to their patients. My psychiatrists were more adamant in prescribing medicine than listening to my thoughts or feelings. They already made a determination of my mental status from what was written even erroneously and at times out of malice by petitioners and believed they were practicing their profession by prescribing medication. I also witnessed no empathy from the psychiatrists and they had a know – it - all attitude with an unbound ego. What happened to truly knowing the patient? Psychiatry has been a major disappointment with doctors spending less than five minutes per appointment while also patients waiting for nearly 40 minutes in the waiting room to see their non-empathetic doctor.

If it wasn't for my court order, I would have left my psychiatrists many years ago. It is unfortunate that psychiatrists prey on the most vulnerable in society so that they can see as many patients as possible in as little time for the greed of billing insurances and making money. I feel like cattle when visiting the psychiatrist, because my thoughts aren't explored yet I'm directed out of the appointment room in a few minute's time with an un-welcomed prescription for medicine.

I have found the field of psychiatry is a struggle to prove my own sanity and even abusive by psychiatrists trying to make me believe something about myself I know not to be true. Psychiatry to me has been abusive, caused mental stress, and duress, because the psychiatrists stated that I fail to see the need for treatment which according to the psychiatrist is a sign of "mental illness!" I'm forced to be stoic when seeing the psychiatrist so that he/she doesn't think I require more medication, but as I stated earlier – times are changing and I'm making my point of view more known. It's bad enough that I'm forced to take medication yet, the thought of being forced to take more medication is a nightmare I wish not to come true.

Writing this book helped clear my thoughts and encouraged me to start a support group for individuals harmed by psychiatry. Even my therapists must learn the importance of empathy and to understand the patient's true reality. I have been a litmus paper for too long determining honest mental health professionals, and now my story must be told. I hope that I succeeded in writing and explaining my objectives in this book, and I'm also optimistic in thinking that we all agree psychiatry needs to change.

Psychiatry has been an unlawful example of medicine gone bad. It seems as though psychiatrists think they're GODS in believing they know how the patient thinks and are omnipotent in understanding the patient's true reality, past, present, or future even without asking the patient relevant questions. The best way to not let a toxic person such as a dishonest psychiatrist ruin your life is to not play with them, however I'm court ordered to but am learning to express myself more. I have no choice but to see my psychiatrist as court ordered and, therefore wrote this book to vent my frustrations and find a form of therapy through writing in expressing my thoughts in the hopes of helping someone cope with their own psychiatric distress, my mental anguish, stress, and duress and change the way psychiatry is practiced.

I further encourage the field of psychiatry to have empathy and understanding of the patient and not "treat" them as though our circumstances and life situations which may have now been resolved, are the same. I furthermore, ask the field of psychiatry to get to know your patients more and use talk therapy/empathy as the major tool in treating the patient and not medicine. In addition, I urge the field of psychiatry to encourage the patient strengthen their communication by socializing more with family and friends in efforts for the patient to be better understood. A better understanding between the patient, family, friends, and medical professionals will also help prevent needless inpatient psychiatric hospitalizations.

Chapter Twenty-Five

Abused by My Petitioners and Psychiatry

It is frustrating knowing that each of the times I was petitioned, the petitioner didn't even speak with me for much time at all! During the 31 years of being wrongfully petitioned, the petitioner didn't speak with me more than a few words in 2-3 week's time before and during each of the petitions! How did the petitioner know what I was actually thinking, if he/she didn't even recently speak with me? – They didn't know what I was thinking and often times my emotional/mental health issues were absolved when the police came to pick me up for a "psychiatric evaluation" which inevitably led to inpatient psychiatric hospitalizations based on the error of physician "playing it safe" and petitioner's "conscience." Often times, my mental health issues were overcome at time of pick-up, but were once again evident after picked up by police officers for a psychiatric evaluation due to feeling like I "must have been a psychiatric patient" and the thought of "behaving like an animal once treated like one." Even now, the petitioners don't talk to me or immediate family any-more than once every two weeks and our conversations only last about a minute! How do these petitioners know me, yet carelessly have made multiple petitions? Once again, they don't know or even knew me, and this form of non-communication yet petition orders was abuse towards me! I never met criteria to be in a psychiatric hospital, because I was never a threat to myself or anyone else but misunderstood due to lack of communication between my petitioners, psychiatry, and myself. I've specifically asked for the petitioners to communicate with me in efforts to better understand each other, yet the petitioners abusively lack to return my favor of more effective communication.

Psychiatry has abused me due to it not exploring my thoughts, yet forcing psychotropic medications on me especially injections! In addition, psychiatry has abused me in regards to forcing me into inpatient psychiatric hospitalizations most often for nearly 30 days and outpatient treatment for nearly two years during each admission! My personal freedom was taken away from me and replaced with tremendous amounts of anguish, stress, distress, and duress! Psychiatry has been a cruel experience for me and I don't condone its existence in the medical field at all until it realizes that the patient's thoughts are most important and must be understood with compassion, patience, empathy, and understanding not through the use of psychotropic medications which debilitate the patient's mind and even cause harmful side-effects.

Chapter Twenty-Six

What "Resolve" Means to Me

Finding resolve with the influences which have caused much grief in my life such as from: being misunderstood, having times of difficulty manifested through psychological issues brought on by a distraught past truly is a blessing. My past difficulties have made me be closer to GOD spiritually and made me realize the greater blessing of living with GOD. My spirituality and being with GOD has taken me away from my turmoil experienced in psychiatry as described in this book.

Resolve to me means rejoicing with GOD over negativity which I've witnessed for many years as described through my events in the mental health system. Rejoicing and finding resolve are two important outcomes I'm thankfully experiencing. Resolve to me, therefore means a stronger being with GOD and rejoice over negativity including my family and friends.

My spirituality and belief in GOD has gotten stronger since all the turmoil and I now understand and have found resolve, because I'm truly happier. My family and friends sense my happiness and they too became to realize the power of being with GOD and having strong spirituality and faith. Every day I wake up thanking GOD for all my family and friends have.

Resolve to me was attained through the understanding that I may not necessarily change people's thoughts or beliefs all the time, but can certainly influence them in a positive way and finding resolve means to me is being positive and rejoicing with GOD, family, and friends. What I have now – stronger spirituality and belief in GOD walking with positive thinking and good spirituality is truly a blessing gained with finding resolve and is something to truly rejoice about and live with each and every day! I therefore, have found an everlasting resolve of which no pill can ever give me, but spirituality and belief in GOD, positive thinking, and surrounding myself with love of being with family and friends manifests. In essence, the negatives strengthened my character, because the negatives were turned into much more stronger positives – much more than I could have imagined and will get even stronger like a snowball getting bigger rolling down a snowy hill but in a positive direction.

Chapter Twenty-Seven

A New Beginning

My undergraduate and graduate study papers focused on a subject close to my heart. How could I not write about a topic that has caused such an enormous amount of misunderstanding, confusion, turmoil, anguish, duress, and stress in my life? I wrote papers while at the university describing my struggles within the mental health system. Specifically, I wrote about strategies used to prevent inpatient psychiatric hospitalizations. I recognized a need to change the mental health system many years ago, and was poised in a position during my studies to actually research and make recommendations to a local community mental health organization. The mental health organization was kind in listening to my concerns. I hope through this book that organizations concerned with mental health will make changes in preventing inpatient psychiatric hospitalizations and realize the power of being more empathetic towards patients.

Without hesitation, I focused much of my independent studies on finding ways to help the mental health system in preventing inpatient psychiatric hospitalizations. I was eager to choose a topic which I believed I could make positive changes and in return would help me by letting the mental health system realize that I may be eccentric at times as we all are, but never needed to be committed into a psychiatric hospital. My field study didn't make its way to completion while in graduate school, because I was withdrawn from the Family Nurse Practitioner program last semester for distributing flyers under people's windshield wipers at my clinical site asking for resolve from the time I was threatened and "let go" from company "Y." It was during that time that I was once again involuntarily admitted into a psychiatric hospital surrounding the stigma of being "mentally ill." My most recent hospitalalization lasted another 30 days, because I refused to take medicine as ordered for the first two weeks of being a patient at the hospital. I refused to take medicine in an effort to make the point that I didn't need to be at the hospital, but was once again misunderstood and stigmatized. My most recent hospitalization inspired me even more to write this book, because I determined "enough is enough" of being wrongfully put through the mental health system. I've been passive for too long and have determined to now make changes and clear my conscience from a system I knew I didn't need to be in as a patient in mental health. I felt enslaved for 30 long years in a system which I fought for the truth I knew, and had tried to make people within the mental health profession aware. I still have resentment until resolve for certain family members for not taking the time to listen to me and try to understand why I thought the way I did, and instead take the easy way out and have me committed once again and forced me into once again taking medicine in an oppressive system - psychiatry. Being a psychiatric patient also carries the stigma of being "mentally ill," which once again, affected my parent time/custody court in a personally negative way with loss of parental Rights for my daughter.

I miss my graduate studies and would be most likely a successful Family Nurse Practitioner, if I wasn't non-empathetically withdrawn from the program. I learned my lesson and have made my thoughts known in writing books. The hard lesson I learned was that stigma and misunderstanding of a person is not a good mix. I therefore made this book to help clarify my own personality and hopefully positively change the mental health system which intermittently left my life and close family and friends devastated and in pieces during the last 30 years. In addition, I hope you found inspiration in reading this book and realizing that if you know something to be true and has bothered you then make positive changes to free yourself from the hardships and lies. I believe GOD has reasons for putting me through the difficult times so that I can inspire others with my success. I truly enjoy being a nurse and have altruistic qualities as in writing this book. I hope you will gain confidence in knowing words can change things as in the hopes of this book making an impact on changing the mental health system. Things are changing in the mental health system as more and more people have had less than "healing" occurrences while being "patients."

It is unfortunate for mental health that the media personifies people with a mental health diagnosis as being the ill people of society. I hope that this book broke down some of the barriers or at least expanded your mind as to other possibilities why people may be caught in the mental health arena.

It's unfortunate all the misunderstanding I've been involved in for the last 30 years of my life, but hope you see that people can fall through the cracks in the mental health system. I have empathy for people that have involuntarily been involved with mental health especially for as long of a period as I have.

Although new technologies have spawned new methods of treatment in psychiatry, we must not forget that people are the ones that suffer if side-effects are present. Psychiatry is a subjective field and should be met with empathy and understanding. I urge the field of psychiatry to listen to your patients and understand that the patient "knows best." I also urge that the system from petition to involuntary commitments into psychiatric hospitals changes more positively with empathy for people such as myself that have "fallen through the cracks" and misunderstood too many times. Psychiatry needs to be a field where the psychiatrist asks the patient questions and attempts to know him/her and not go for the quick fix and prescribe medicine – having empathy is the key to understanding and a good start.

About the Author

My name is John Peter Veremis and I'm empathetic of other people's thoughts and feelings.I enjoy drawing, candle making, exercising, Wellness, and lead a relatively healthy life. I'm also proactive and enjoy encouraging others to also lead healthy mentally, physically, and spiritual lives. I have two wonderful children and am living with my mother enjoying all that she teaches us in her elderly years.

www.ingramcontent.com/pod-product-compliance
Lightning Source LLC
LaVergne TN
LVHW090416210926
848480LV00002B/582
* 9 7 9 8 2 3 0 8 7 7 2 8 8 *